Saundra
Thompson
382-6759

SECOND EDITION

Creative Aerobic Fitness:
A guide to active living

Robin D. Reese, Ph.D.

Jayne A. Willett, M.A., ATC

Jennifer K. Park, B.S.

Rosie Castañeda, M.S.

D1528937

KENDALL/HUNT PUBLISHING COMPANY
4050 Westmark Drive   Dubuque, Iowa 52002

Copyright © 1988, 1995 by Kendall/Hunt Publishing Company

ISBN 0-8403-9884-0

All rights reserved. No part of this publication
may be reproduced, stored in a retrieval system, or
transmitted, in any form or by any means, elec-
tronic, mechanical, photocopying, recording, or
otherwise, without the prior written permission of
the copyright owner.

Printed in the United States of America
10   9   8   7   6   5   4   3   2   1

Contents

Preface

Creative Aerobic Fitness: A guide to active living is in sync with the fitness movement currently sweeping our country. Many young adults, concerned with looking good and feeling healthy, are joining fitness clubs and/or registering for classes at their local college or university. The purpose of this text is to help those young people, as well as older adults, better understand the road to aerobic fitness so that they might avoid bumps and potholes, choose the best individual route, navigate correctly, arrive safely at their destination, and stay there—for a lifetime.

College texts for the aerobic enthusiast are often too broad or too narrow. That is, they attempt to cover all sports and activities that strengthen the cardiorespiratory system, or they choose a single one; i.e., aerobic dance. *Creative Aerobic Fitness: A guide to active living* goes beyond aerobic dance. It recognizes the variety of popular activities that can be performed by individuals or a group to promote aerobic conditioning and total fitness. Whether high impact, low impact, integrated aerobics, stepping, sculpting, walking or sliding, the limits of safe and effective aerobic fitness is bounded only by the imagination of the instructor and the preference of the participants. Students able to experience and practice each style of movement should be able to develop a repertoire of activities compatible with their talent and interests. We believe that students who participate in activities that are fun and engaging will stay on the road to good health.

Creative Aerobic Fitness: A guide to active living is divided into four parts and thirteen chapters. The first part is introductory in nature. Chapters 1, 2 and 3 let the reader know what to expect, what to be wary of, and how to get started. This section also addresses the role of motivation in the development and maintenance of an active lifestyle.

The second section provides the ways and means to total fitness, with the chapters sequenced in an order that parallels their introduction in a typical class. Chapter 4 acquaints the reader with the components of health-related physical fitness, motor ability, good posture and the correct way to breathe during exercise, while Chapter 5 recommends pre and post tests for selected fitness components so that improvement can be objectively measured and goals established. Chapter 6 stresses the importance of a rhythmic warm up, followed by safe static stretches. Chapter 7 explores the prescription for aerobic exercise that specifies the frequency, intensity, duration and mode that are necessary for full realization of the physiological and psychological benefits attributed to aerobic exercise. Chapter 8 introduces the reader to creative aerobic movements, distinguishing between impact variations, intensity modifications, and choreography options. Chapter 9 concentrates on cooling down. This includes bringing the heart rate down slowly, increasing the endurance and flexibility of specific muscle groups and relaxing the total body before leaving class. Chapter 10 discusses the options provided by variety training. Presented here is information about supplemental exercises, including fitness walking, rope jumping, water exercise, step aerobics and sliding.

The third part is devoted to weight management. Chapter 11 provides the reader with a thorough understanding of the principles of good nutrition, while Chapter 12 explores the interaction between diet and exercise with an emphasis on safely losing unwanted fat. The fourth and final section consists of a single chapter that deals with the recognition, and most importantly, the prevention and care of common aerobic injuries, should there be any.

The appendices are geared specifically for college classes but can be used by anyone looking for program structure and feedback. Appendix A assists in establishing guidelines for individual exercise participation by identifying personal health history, present level of conditioning and prescribed exercise intensity. Appendix B is a means of exploring program options related to both content and structure. Using the tools provided here, exercise participants gain critical feedback regarding the effectiveness of different types of workouts. The use of these tools is beneficial to anyone trying to develop responsibility towards their own health and fitness.

CHAPTER 1

Aerobic Exercise

You don't have to be thin to be fit. You don't have to be beautiful to be radiant. People who are "in shape" create an aura around them that is simply captivating. To others they possess energy and carry themselves with confidence. To themselves they feel good about who they are and where they are going. Fit individuals have discovered a key, and use it regularly to unlock doors that might otherwise keep them from realizing their full potential. They have found that regular activity builds their mind and body. They have discovered aerobic exercise.

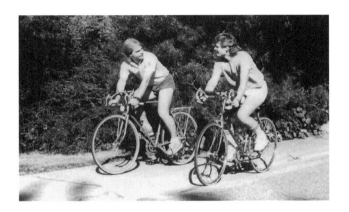

AEROBIC EXERCISE DEFINED

The term aerobic means "with oxygen." Oxygen contributes to the production of energy for muscle contraction during aerobic exercise. **Aerobic exercise** is *rigorous physical activity that utilizes oxygen for a sustained period of time without rest intervals.* Some of the more popular forms of aerobic exercise include:

- aerobic dance & rhythmic movement
- brisk walking, jogging & running
- cardiovascular machines (treadmill, stepper, ergometer, etc.)
- circuit training
- cross country skiing
- cycling
- hiking & backpacking
- jumping rope
- rowing
- skating
- sliding
- stepping & stair climbing
- swimming & water exercise

CREATIVE AEROBIC EXERCISE

Creative aerobic exercise *includes those popular forms of aerobic activity that can be performed to music by a group or an individual using minimal equipment.* In addition to enhancing fitness and health, classes in creative aerobic fitness are designed to promote social interaction, fun and enjoyment. A primary goal is to demonstrate that getting in shape and staying in shape can actually be fun. Select your favorite creative aerobic activities from any of the following skills and movement styles:

- low, high or integrated impact aerobics
- freestyle, choreographed or add-on patterns
- walking, water exercise or jumping rope
- sculpting, stepping or sliding.

The variety of the activity is limited only by the imagination and creativity of the instructor, equipment availability and safety concerns.

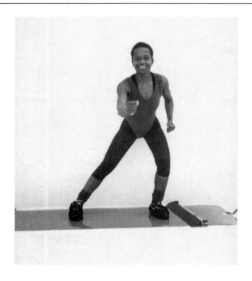

A NATIONAL PRESCRIPTION FOR AEROBIC EXERCISE

If you're not already active there are many reasons you should start an exercise program now. In 1990, the Federal Department of Health and Human Services published national health recommendations to all Americans. In the report entitled *Healthy People 2000* an active lifestyle and regular exercise are viewed as the number one priority of health promotion.

Why all the fuss? Coronary heart disease (CHD) is the leading cause of all deaths in the United States and has been for several decades. Research has shown that regular physical activity reduces the risk of CHD. That is, prevention of cardiovascular disease has been scientifically related to quality exercise, as well as to a good diet. Through regular aerobic exercise you not only improve your fitness, but contribute to your long term health.

An active lifestyle starts with selecting an aerobic activity from the previous list and following these research based guidelines:

—exercise at least three times per week

—exercise at an individually prescribed intensity

—exercise at least:
  ten minutes two or more times daily for minimum benefits
  or
  20–60 minutes in a continuous session for maximum benefits

Sound easy? It really can be quite simple, once you realize you control and determine your own lifestyle. In chapters 2 and 7 you will learn more about developing and maintaining an exercise program that meets your own needs.

BENEFITS OF REGULAR AEROBIC EXERCISE

The benefits that can be derived from regular participation in a safe and correctly prescribed aerobic exercise program are truly amazing. Developing fitness not only contributes to your physical health but helps you look and feel better.

Physiological Benefits

Increasing **aerobic capacity,** *the ability to take in, transport, and utilize oxygen,* by increasing the demand placed on the cardiorespiratory system with vigorous aerobic exercise results in a significant "training effect". The **training effect,** or *beneficial physiological changes that will occur when a program is continuous for a period of 8–12 weeks,* include:

1. Stronger respiratory muscles and increased lung capacity. The ability to inspire greater amounts of oxygen into the lungs results in less strain on the heart.

2. A stronger heart with a corresponding increase in stroke volume. **Stroke volume** *refers to the amount of blood pumped with each beat.* This results in a lower **resting heart rate** or *number of times the heart beats in one minute while the body is at rest.* Resting heart rates may range from 40–100 beats per minute. Seventy-two is considered average. An aerobically active person often has a resting heart rate under 60 beats per minute, while a sedentary person typically has one that is much higher. A low resting heart rate is desirable because it gives the heart muscle more time to rest between beats.

3. Improved **cardiac output** or *total amount of blood the heart pumps and circulates in one minute.* At rest, a strong, trained heart distributes the same blood volume per minute as an untrained heart, but it does so with fewer and stronger contractions. During vigorous exercise, however, a strong trained heart is capable of circulating a much greater volume of blood per minute than an untrained heart.

4. Improved circulation through expansion (vasodilation) and contraction (vasoconstriction) of the blood vessels.

5. Lower blood pressure for some individuals as a result of improved circulation.

6. An increase in **high density lipoproteins (HDL).** These *small, high density, protective protein molecules carry excess fats, including cholesterol, from the bloodstream to the liver for elimination.* A lower concentration of fat in the bloodstream results in less blockage or damage to artery walls, significantly reducing the risk of coronary heart disease.

7. Increased sensitivity to insulin and lowered blood sugar levels. This is especially important for Type II diabetics whose bodies while producing insulin no longer respond effectively. Their body literally becomes insulin resistant. This problem can be related to hereditary, pregnancy, aging, and/or weight gain. Regard-

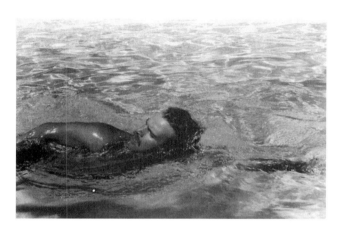

less of its cause, insulin sensitivity can be increased through low intensity to moderate levels of exercise and a controlled diet. (Pregnant women who develop Type II diabetes should exercise under a doctor's supervision.)

8. Increased bone density (stronger bones) that may prevent the onset of osteoporosis later in life.

9. Improved muscle tone and endurance.

10. Positive changes in body composition (less fat, more muscle).

11. Improved weight control.

12. A more regular elimination of solid wastes.

13. Ability to fall asleep more quickly and sleep more soundly.

14. Reduced risk of cardiovascular disease.

15. Possible delay in the aging process.

Psychological Benefits

Once you have achieved the training effect, you will begin to experience some positive psychological changes. It is really these changes that are responsible for the "radiance" and feeling of well being discussed earlier in this chapter. These include, but are not limited to:

1. Increased energy and enthusiasm for living life to its fullest.

2. Improved mental capabilities such as concentration and self discipline.

3. The ability to manage stress more effectively.

4. Increased self-confidence.

5. Enhanced self-concept and self-image leading to more positive feelings about yourself and eventually a more positive attitude toward others.

People who have committed themselves to a regular program of aerobic exercise will tell you that all of the benefits listed in this section are real and attainable. It is up to you to decide if they are the kinds of changes you want to experience in your life. If so, it is going to take time, effort and commitment.

MAKING A COMMITMENT FOR LIFE

The prescription for aerobic exercise is similar to a prescription for antibiotics. Both are used to promote health. While one fights infection, the other promotes fitness. However, there is an important difference. Unlike a prescription for penicillin, which is taken for a relatively short time, the prescription for aerobic exercise never expires. To continue receiving the physiological and psychological benefits of exercise you must maintain an active lifestyle.

Exercise isn't something that you do sporadically just because you feel energetic or depressed. Exercise isn't something you do each spring as bathing suit season approaches or the day after Thanksgiving because you ate too much food. Nor is exercise something you can abandon periodically because you just don't have time. There are many reasons we start fitness programs and there are even more reasons we stop or get side-tracked.

The simple truth remains that physical fitness, once developed, can only be maintained through ongoing exercise. Activity performed regularly each week involves nothing less than a lifetime commitment. The quality of your life depends on it!

SUMMARY

Getting in shape and staying in shape can be enjoyable. It can also change your life. Creative aerobic exercise, performed regularly and continuously with your heart rate at a predetermined level will, after 8–12 weeks, yield multiple physiological and psychological benefits. These benefits are worth the effort and will reinforce your continued commitment to a healthier and happier life.

GLOSSARY

Aerobic Capacity—the maximum rate at which one's body can take in, transport and utilize oxygen.

Aerobic Conditioning—the process and results of aerobic exercise may also be referred to as aerobic training, cardiovascular conditioning, cardiovascular training, cardiorespiratory endurance or aerobic endurance.

Aerobic Exercise—rigorous physical activity that challenges the cardiorespiratory system to supply adequate oxygen to sustain performance for long periods of time.

Cardiac Output—the total amount of blood the heart pumps and circulates in one minute.

Creative Aerobic Exercise—aerobic exercise performed indoors to popular music without expensive equipment that promotes creativity, challenge, fitness and fun.

High Density Lipoprotein (HDL)—a small protein molecule that carries fat and cholesterol from the bloodstream and is thought to provide some protection against coronary heart disease.

Low Density Lipoprotein (LDL)—a medium-sized protein molecule that may be deposited on the artery walls and increase the risk of coronary heart disease.

Resting Heart Rate—the number of times the heart beats in one minute while the body is at rest.

Stroke Volume—the amount of blood pumped out of the heart with each beat.

Training Effect—beneficial physiological changes that occur in the body when a prescribed aerobic program has been adhered to for a period of 8–12 weeks.

REFERENCES

Åstrand, P. (1992). "Why exercise?" *Medicine and Science in Sports and Exercise, 24* (2), 153–162.

Blair, S. N. (1993). 1993 C. H. McCloy research lecture: Physical activity, physical fitness and health. *Research Quarterly for Exercise and Sport, 64* (4), 365–376.

McGinnis, J. M. (1992). The public health burden of a sedentary lifestyle. *Medicine and Science in Sports and Exercise, 24* (6) S196–S200.

Sherman, W. M. & Albright, A. (1992). Exercise and Type II diabetes. *Sports Science Exchange, 4* (37).

Sopko, G., Obarzanek, E., & Stone, E. (1992). Overview of the National Heart, Lung and Blood Institute Workshop on physical activity and cardiovascular health. *Medicine and Science in Sports and Exercise, 24* (6), S192–S195.

Young, D. R. & Steinhardt, M. A. (1993). The importance of physical fitness versus physical activity for coronary and artery disease risk factors: A cross-sectional analysis. *Research Quarterly for Exercise and Sport, 64* (4), 377–384.

Individuality is to be preserved and respected everywhere.
–Jean Paul Richter Titan, 1803

CHAPTER 2

Individualizing Your Program

Adopting an active lifestyle requires ongoing motivation and the courage to make a commitment. The requirements may seem overwhelming. Just considering this endeavor means putting your ego on the line. Fear of failure is not an uncommon concern. You think "is this something I can really do?"; "what if I don't like exercising?". Everyone's expectations and reactions to exercise are unique. Inherent differences in physical ability, performance, and enjoyment demand an individualized approach even within group activities. The need to modify, adapt, and substitute exercises to meet the individual needs of each participant is crucial to developing a successful program. Acknowledging the risks that exist and understanding yourself, your limitations, and what you can realistically accomplish may help reduce your fears. Recognizing the importance of motivation is also crucial for success. The purpose of this chapter is to identify and discuss the special concerns and considerations that are universal in nature and those that are more personal. Not every topic will apply to you, but the knowledge gained from reading each may benefit someone you know or assist you at a later time.

GENERAL HEALTH CONSIDERATIONS

Risk Know

The American College of Sports Medicine identifies five major **coronary risk factors:** *diagnosed high blood pressure, elevated serum cholesterol, diabetes, smoking, and a family history of coronary artery disease.* If you are a man over 40 years old or a woman above the age of 50, "apparently healthy" with no special medical considerations or restrictions then you are generally considered safe to begin a moderate exercise program. However, anyone, regardless of age, exhibiting two or more coronary risk factors or who displays "symptoms of possible cardiopulmonary or metabolic disease" are considered at "higher risk". These individuals should

receive a medical exam and diagnostic exercise test prior to engaging in a vigorous exercise program. A moderate exercise program may be initiated if the activity is non-competitive, progresses slowly, and is of low to moderate intensity (ACSM, 1991).

These recommendations are made for your protection. A person at higher risk should adopt a vigorous exercise program only with the assistance and approval of their physician. While apparently healthy individuals are encouraged to monitor their blood pressure and cholesterol and seek regular physical examinations, these concerns should not preclude involvement in a regular exercise program.

Students enrolled in creative aerobic fitness may be asked to complete a medical profile (Appendix A). University students generally have access to the campus health center and may be able to arrange for a physical exam at little or no cost. Check with your instructor for details.

ABNORMAL CARDIOVASCULAR RESPONSES DURING EXERCISE

In general, individuals considered to be in good health need not be concerned with developing abnormal heart responses during exercise. Heart complications could, however, arise without warning. If any of the following symptoms appear during exercise, and/or after the exercise has ceased, inform your instructor immediately and seek medical advice:

- Tightness or pain in center of chest
- Radiating pain down left arm
- Staggering or persistent unsteadiness
- Unusual or severe fatigue
- Mental confusion
- Fainting

- Sudden rapid heart beats
- Irregular pulse
- Fluttering heart beats
- Sudden change in pulse rate from very high to very low

THE OLDER ADULT

At what age does a person become an "older adult"? The issue is still being debated. The biggest argument is over the difference between chronological aging (how old you are) and physiological aging (how efficient your body is). Chronological age is a convenient measure that is often used to categorize normal growth and adaptation. In children we use age to predict the development of normal behaviors and motor skills. We have different expectations of a seven-year-old than we do a two-year-old or a twelve-year-old. However, this has never been as easy nor as accurate at the other end of the aging continuum. What differences do we expect from someone who is 60, or 65, or 70? While we can observe and even predict certain changes in physiological function over time, the problem is that we are unable to accurately establish when these changes will occur. Since age may not be the best way to evaluate the needs of an older adult, we will describe changes observed as a result of normal aging and recommend that individuals and their instructors use these as guidelines for making program modifications.

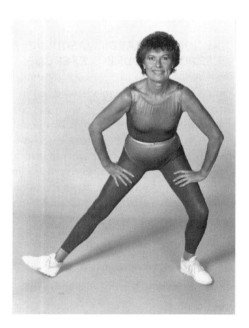

Muscular strength and flexibility decline with age. A measurable decrease in bone density leading to osteoporosis (breaking down of the bone tissue) has also been observed in aging individuals, especially among post-menopausal women. On a positive note, the training effect has been observed in individuals of all ages, indicating that with regular exercise muscular strength and flexibility can and will improve. Bones respond to weight bearing exercise, such as aerobic dance, by acquiring more calcium and becoming more dense. In addition to regular exercise, people of all ages require intake of dietary calcium to develop and maintain strong bones.

While no one is ever really too old to exercise, there are some things to consider before plunging in. It is now a commonly accepted practice among fitness experts to recommend a physical exam prior to participation in an exercise program with annual follow-up exams to ensure continued good health. Let your doctor help you choose the best program based on your needs and physical condition. Age is not a good reason to deny yourself the opportunity to engage in an exercise program, but it is a reason to visit your doctor. Remember, "older" is usually associated with "wiser". So, be the wiser and see your doctor.

FEMALE CONCERNS

Breast Soreness

Many women experience breast soreness during exercise. This discomfort can be minimized by wearing a snugly fitting bra or a special "exercise" bra. The exercise bra can be purchased at most large department stores and/or sports shops. It is recommended that some kind of support be worn not only to reduce the discomfort but to avoid stress to breast tissue.

The Menstrual Cycle

The menstrual cycle has been used repeatedly as an excuse to avoid exercise. Concerns range from real physical discomfort to unfounded fear. Many myths about exercise and the menstrual cycle have previously kept girls and women from exercising. The rumor that exercise or any physical activity can cause the uterus to drop or even fall out is simply not true.

Menstrual "cramps" or dysmenorrhea are experienced by many women. Exercise has been associated with relief of monthly symptoms for some women, but not all. It is believed that the increased oxygen flow throughout the body during aerobic activity serves to stimulate the system, minimizing discomfort.

A program of regular aerobic exercise may or may not affect a woman's menstrual cycle. Changes may result in one of the following: a more regular cycle; oligomenorrhea, a markedly diminished flow and/or an irregular cycle; ovulatory dysfunction, delay or absence of ovulation even with normal menses; or amenorrhea, an abnormal absence of the cycle. There is ongoing disagreement and speculation among researchers as to the cause of these menstrual changes. Among the reasons previously investigated are psychological stress, premature menopause, diet and/or inadequate body fat. None of these conditions have been scientifically linked with menstrual disorders despite the attention they have received (Loucks, Vaitukaitis, Cameron, Rogol, Skrinar, Warren, Kendrick, & Limacher, 1992).

There is still relatively little known about the short and long term effects of increased physical training on the female reproductive function. Whatever the undetermined cause of missed periods and/or absent ovulation, the potential development of osteoporosis is a direct consequence. Osteoporosis, is generally a concern of older, post menopausal women and is often managed through hormone therapy. For young women who do not have their menstrual irregularities treated the risk of osteoporosis may go undiagnosed and, therefore, pose an undetected threat to overall health. Another consequence of missed periods and abnormal ovulation is infertility. The chance of becoming pregnant with either of these conditions is minimal.

Perhaps the alteration in the menstrual pattern is a temporary adjustment that will reverse itself in time. This question is still under investigation. None-the-less, missed or absent periods are not normal. While many women may jump for joy that the cycle has stopped, there are too many unanswered questions and unfortunate consequences to warrant excitement. Clearly, menstrual irregularity or dysfunction should not be ignored. This condition should be carefully evaluated by a physician.

Pregnancy and Exercise

If you become pregnant, whether you have been exercising or not, your doctor needs to be notified. Generally, if you have been involved in a regular exercise program, you may continue with some modifications. Changes from a regular exercise to a prenatal program involves lowering the training heart rate zone, minimizing elevation of body temperature, and after the first trimester, avoiding supine exercises. Supine refers to laying on your back. A **supine exercise** is any movement performed in this position, including abdominal curls, pelvic tilts and many leg exercises. Other exercises should be substituted to work these target areas. The specific modifications will be recommended by your doctor. Exercise guidelines developed by the American College of Obstetricians and Gynecologists will help your physician select the appropriate mode of activity, frequency, intensity and duration.

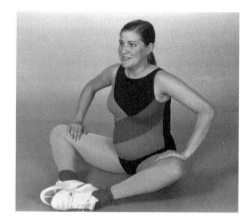

ORTHOPEDIC CONCERNS

There are numerous orthopedic injuries or conditions which may affect you and alter the way in which you can exercise or carry out the tasks of daily living. Common **acute injuries** (sudden onset, usually short in duration) affecting muscles, joints and bones include: muscle strains, ligament sprains, cartilage tears, joint separations or dislocations and fractures to bones. These types of injuries may occur at any time as a result of a sudden abnormal motion, whether exercising or not. **Chronic injuries** (gradual onset, long duration) such as tendinitis, low back pain and stress fractures are usually the result of overuse and are often complicated by musculoskeletal malalignment and/or structural imbalance. Proper medical care is necessary and a must if one is to return to normal daily activities, including exercise. More details relative to specific injury recognition and care are given in Chapter 13.

If you have sustained an injury or experience discomfort in a particular joint you may need to modify your exercise program to allow that joint and surrounding musculature to adapt to the new stresses. In addition, you may find it necessary to omit certain movement patterns from your exercise program altogether. Even those of you who have never experienced injury may find that you are not capable of performing certain movement patterns without discomfort. Each of you has a unique musculoskeletal structure with varying degrees of strength and flexibility that directly influences your functional capabilities. You may have some limitations and should learn to recognize and work within those limitations in an effort to prevent injury.

Common aerobic injuries may be prevented with a basic understanding of how the human body manages external or incoming forces. First, imagine the body as a huge shock absorber. Each step, hop or jump creates a shock wave. In an effort to dissipate the shock wave, the musculoskeletal system acts to distribute the forces throughout the body. Landing forces are absorbed by shock absorbing structures such as the muscles of the lower extremity, the menisci (cartilages of the knee), the intervertebral disks of the spine (in particular the lumbar spine) and by the bones. When structural malalignment is present and/or an individual is carrying an excess of body weight, the shock absorbing system is subject to breakdown. During activities such as run-

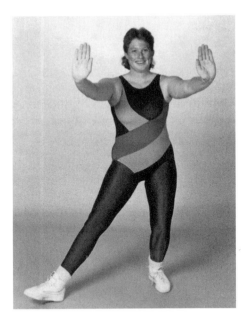

ning and jumping, landing forces have been recorded in the order of three to six times the body weight. When these forces are coupled with malalignment and/or excess weight, the stress often exceeds the critical limits of the shock absorbing structures in the body and injury is the result. Thus,

shock absorption is a major concern in injury prevention.

Sports medicine professionals (Doctors, Biomechanists, Physical Therapists, Athletic Trainers, Biomedical Engineers, etc.) have been studying methods to reduce the impact forces in a variety of sport activities for some time. The athletic shoe has received most of the attention since the beginning of the running boom. Researchers have learned a lot about the shock absorbing characteristics of hundreds of materials and have designed shoes according to the specific directional movement patterns of a sport, as well as the type and amount of impact forces delivered to the body while engaged in that sport. Selecting proper footwear for participation in creative aerobic fitness will be discussed in Chapter 3.

Another important aspect of injury prevention is the workout surface or exercise floor. Exercise floors used for creative aerobic exercise vary from carpet covered cement, to wooden gym floors to the new spring loaded floors. As a result of an increase in the injury rate among aerobic enthusiasts, an effort has been made to control the type of surface used for exercise. The latest innovation is the spring loaded floor, either wooden or lightly carpeted. Recent research has shown a favorable decline in the injury rate for lower leg and knee pain as a result of the new spring type floors. Unfortunately, these floors are quite costly and not available for every club, studio or school setting. In some school settings gymnastic or wrestling mats may substitute for quality flooring, but participants trade the cushioning provided by the mat for a lack of stability. Using this type of surface may lead to knee or ankle discomfort. The typical college surface is the standard wooden gym floor. This is not the worst choice for aerobic exercise but certainly warrants a good pair of shoes.

Lower leg pain (shin splints) and knee pain are reportedly at the top of the injury list among aerobics enthusiasts. These injuries are directly influenced by the type of shoe and surface quality. Fortunately, bones, muscles and tendons will generally adapt to the stresses and become stronger over time. The key is to start slowly, progress gradually, and use good common sense.

Additional guidelines for injury prevention include a proper warm-up and cool-down, plenty of water before, during and after class and a well balanced diet. Nutritional deficits and dehydration can result in muscle cramping, constant soreness and undue fatigue, all of which may serve as precursors to serious injury. Listen to your body and learn how to make it the best it can be—safely.

SELF-IMAGE

The physical exam is complete and your doctor applauds your involvement in regular exercise. You're advised by your doctor and instructor to begin slowly, listen to your body and don't over do it! These are sensible guidelines that anyone can follow. Yet you have lingering doubts; feelings that hold you back. Are you concerned with how you will look in exercise attire? Are you self-conscious of your arms, thighs, or abdomen; your entire body? Maybe you're one of only a few men in a class dominated by women. Perhaps some of the movements make you feel awkward. Regardless of the exact nature of your concern, you are anxious about what others will think. Can you measure up to the expectations of your classmates or instructor? Perhaps the real issue is measuring up to your own expectations!

This is a typical scenario experienced by men and women of all ages. It is surprising how many people are uncomfortable with their physical appearance or self-conscious about the way they move. While there are not enough pages in this text to discuss self-image in detail, we can say that regular exercise has been associated with the development of a positive self-image. If exercise can have a positive effect on self-image, confidence and ultimately on self-concept, it is probably worth trying.

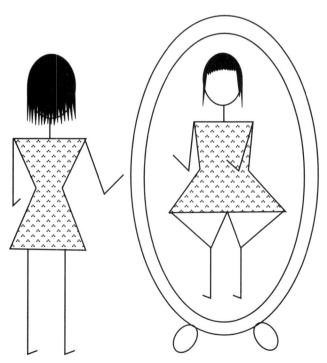

Body-image is how we perceive ourselves to look. We may have a distorted view of our image and feel negatively towards our body.

Perhaps just as critical as the development of a positive self-image is the acceptance of the body you were born with. Exercise can change your body composition, add definition to your arms and legs and lower body fat (see chapter 5). However, no amount of exercise can alter your basic body structure (see chapter 12). Many of us look in the mirror and are disappointed with what we see. We have been overwhelmed with images of what advertising executives deem the perfect body. Chances are we don't look like the women and men on magazine covers and no amount of exercise will change that. Whether the concern is a disproportional body or being over or under weight, the image we see in that mirror often centers on our perceived shortcomings. The next time you look in the mirror instead of comparing yourself to a model or focusing on areas needing improvement, find those features that flatter. Remember, attractiveness is not based solely on physical attributes but inner qualities as well. Poise and self-confidence are attractive.

MOTIVATION

The term motivation is from the Latin term *movere*—which literally means to move. Being motivated implies some type of aroused state leading to an action or behavior. We have all been motivated to take actions; however, many of us lose our initial interest and eventually stop. Consider all of the projects you have started and not completed. Specifically think of each time you've initiated an exercise program or weight loss diet and then given up. Was motivation a factor? Making permanent changes in our lifestyle requires ongoing motivation. There are several strategies to staying motivated.

First you need to understand two important facts about behavior modification and lifestyle development:

1. Education is an important factor changing behavior

2. Knowledge alone does not elicit desired behavior.

Unfortunately this means that even after people know that exercise and diet are important to good health and quality of life, many individuals will still have difficulty acting on this knowledge.

The secret ingredient to developing and maintaining an active lifestyle consists of the *right motivation* and the perception that an individual can *control their behavior*.

CONSIDER THIS
STARTLING
OBSERVATION:

> The drop out rate from cardiac rehabilitation programs has been reported to be almost 50% (Franklin, 1988; Oldridge, 1984), and these are people whose lives depend on exercise!!!!

Taking Responsibility for Your Actions

What is the difference between those who disrupt their exercise schedule because of other priorities and those who just stop exercising? Could the distinction be attitude and self-concept? Those who define themselves as "active" will do so even when not exercising. Taking vacations, responding to emergency situations, even resting an injury will not make them feel like an exercise dropout. They will plan and look forward to returning to regular exercise. On the other hand, those who hesitate to consider themselves active after taking a day off or those who refer to themselves as exercise dropouts are destined to fail. Lifestyle is as much about attitude as it is about actions.

Now and then everyone takes time off from exercise, but the self-discipline that must accompany an active lifestyle helps them make the decision to return to exercise as soon as possible. Self-discipline is a valuable quality. A quality that we all have to some degree, but one which we don't always apply to sensible eating and regular exercise. Self-discipline is the responsibility you take over your actions. It is the characteristic you use to make yourself study, attend class, show up for work on time, and even exercise. Self-discipline is related to your self-image and past experience. If you consider yourself a success, then self-discipline will be used to actualize that image of yourself. If your past experience with exercise has been less than successful, imagine another challenging situation which has brought you accomplishment and adopt the attitude that helped you persevere.

By taking responsibility for your actions, but not punishing yourself or overreacting to unwanted behavior, you can elicit desired outcomes. For example, you want to exercise three times per week but find that studying for a midterm will interfere with a regular exercise session. As a responsible student you choose to study for the exam. As a responsible exercise participant you select to take 10 minute breaks and climb the stairs in the library, perform two sets of crunches, and/or stretch in your seat. These small fitness sessions not only help your body, but provide you with an effective study tool. Structured mental breaks actually help you decrease physical and mental fatigue, allowing you to focus and improve comprehension.

There are always situations that interfere with exercise and a variety of circumstances that should take priority over activity, including illness, injury, emergencies, and many personal and professional commitments. When you have the stomach flu, the responsible action is to forego exercise for rest. However, you need to be sure that you don't over react with guilt or other types of self-punishment. Taking a few days or more off from exercise is at times unavoidable and at other times necessary. The important thing to remember is that your self-image should not suffer just because you're not exercising. It's all about perspective. Don't consider yourself a dropout statistic or a sedentary person just because you haven't been especially active. Consider yourself an exercise participant on a well deserved vacation, an active person taking time off because of other responsibilities, or a fit person taking the time off to let an injury heal. You can control your perception of yourself. Don't let inactivity keep you from returning to exercise.

Motivation and Movement

The secret ingredients to developing and maintaining an active lifestyle consist of the perception that *you are an active person* and a focus on *the appropriate motivation*. Two basic types of MOTIVATION have been identified: *internal*, from within, and *external*, from the outside. In exercise, internal motivation can lead to participating in activities that you enjoy, that make you feel good, or that elicit a sense of success. In exercise external motivation can lead to participating in activities that you think will help you lose weight, look better, or that have been recommended to you by a friend.

Rewards stemming from *internal motivation* are usually related to the process of the activity and result in immediate gratification. With *external motivation* performing the activity itself does not inherently reward the participant; the rewards tend to be delayed or may never be fully realized. The nature of this motivation centers around some outcome or product that is usually unrelated to the activity itself. The key to exercise adherence is to locate your own internal motivation. Find activities that provide you with a sincere sense of enjoyment. Emphasize the process rather than the product of movement. Some benefits of exercise (weight loss, improved fitness) tend to be "long term" rather than immediate. These are very good reasons to exercise but may not provide you with the motivation you need to continue a program.

Initially focusing on long-term goals can lead to excessive behavior, which in respect to exercise means doing too much too soon. **Excessive exercise will not** speed up permanent results, but more likely lead to mental and physical BURN-OUT. If you are new to aerobic exercise, it is important to find *activities* that provide immediate gratification (something enjoyed simply through the activity). Notice that the word activities is plural. Having a single mode of exercise to choose from may eventually lead to boredom. Program variety will relieve physical and mental overtraining. Consider emphasizing the process of the activity (sense of involvement, joy of movement, etc.) rather than the product (weight loss, or reduced blood pressure).

Many of the training effects of exercise (improved aerobic capacity, increased stamina, etc.) can be realized after 8–10 weeks of a regular cardiovascular program. However, the larger the goal the more time training will take. Long-term goals should be accompanied by smaller short-term goals. A short-term goal should be a measurable change or modification that can be reasonably achieved within a few weeks or a month. Goal setting will be discussed in more detail in chapter 5.

SUMMARY

The purpose of this chapter was to highlight and discuss special concerns shared by new and long term exercise enthusiasts alike. Many of the most commonly asked questions have been answered, providing you with increased awareness and a more informed approach toward understanding and managing various exercise related concerns. In addition to physical concerns, motivation and self-image are individual factors that will affect your exercise participation. Learn to be comfortable with your body, seek out activities you enjoy, and accept your limitations as well as your potential. If you have concerns that are not addressed in this chapter, you are encouraged to consult with your instructor.

GLOSSARY

Amenorrhea—the abnormal absence or suppression of the menstrual cycle in females who were previously menstrual.

Coronary Risk Factors—individual characteristics that have been identified as contributing to heart disease: the five primary factors include high blood pressure, elevated serum cholesterol, diabetes, smoking, and a family history of coronary artery disease.

Dysmenorrhea—menstrual cramping and discomfort.

Long-Term Goals—accomplishments that may take several months or even a year to achieve.

Motivation—the desire to act or move; an important factor in maintaining an exercise program and an active lifestyle.

Oligomenorrhea—a markedly diminished menstrual flow and/or irregular cycles (used interchangeably with the term irregular).

Osteoporosis—a breaking down of the bones due to demineralization; seen mostly in the elderly or in younger women who exhibit menstrual irregularity over extended periods of time.

Short-Term Goals—accomplishments that can be achieved in a relatively small period of time; those related to exercise may take a few weeks or a month.

Supine Exercise—any physical activity performed while laying on the back.

REFERENCES

Clapp, III, J. F., Rokey, R., Treadway, J. L., Carpenter, M. W., Artal, R. M., Warrnes, C. (1992). Exercise and Pregnancy. *Medicine and Science in Sports and Exercise, 24* (6), Supplement, S294–S299.

Franklin, B. A. (1988). Program factors that influence exercise adherence: Practical adherence skills for the clinical staff. In R. K. Dishman (Ed.), *Exercise adherence: It's impact on public health* (pp. 237–258). Champaign, IL: Human Kinetics.

Horn, T. S. (1992). *Advances in Sport Psychology.* Champaign, IL: Human Kinetics.

King, A. C., Blair, S. N., Bild, D. E., Dishman, R. K., Dubbert, P. M., Marcus, B. H., Oldridge, N. B., Paffenbarger, Jr., R. S., Powell, K. E., Yeager, K. K. (1992). Determinants of physical activity and interventions in adults. *Medicine and Science in Sports and Exercise, 24* (6), Supplement, S221–233.

Loucks, A. B., Vaitukaitis, J., Cameron, J. L., Rogol, A. D., Skrinar, G., Warren, M. P., Kendrick, J., & Limacher, M. C. (1992). The reproductive system and exercise in women. *Medicine and Science in Sports and Exercise, 24* (6), Supplement, S288–S292.

Oldridge, N. B. (1984). Compliance and dropout rate in cardiac exercise rehabilitation. *Journal of Cardiac Rehabilitation, 4,* 166–177.

Pivarnik, J. M., Ayres, N. A., Mauer, M. B., Cotton, D. B., Kirshon, B., & Dildy, G. A. (1993). Effects of maternal aerobic fitness on the cardiorespiratory response to exercise. *Medicine and Science in Sports and Exercise, 25* (9), 993–998.

Rejeski, W. J. & Kenney, E. A. (1988). *Fitness Motivation: Preventing Participant Fallout.* Champaign, IL: Life Enhancement Publications.

Wankel, L. M. (1987). Enhancement motivation or involvement in voluntary exercise programs. In M. L. Maehr (Ed.), *Advances in motivation and achievement: Enhancing motivation* (vol. 5, pp. 239–286). Greenwich, CT: JAI Press.

Willis, J. D., Campbell, L. F. (1992). *Exercise Psychology.* Champaign, IL: Human Kinetics.

Distance is nothing; it is only the first step that is difficult.
–Marie Anne du Deffand, 1763

CHAPTER 3

Getting Started

By now you should be fully aware of the benefits and concerns associated with aerobic exercise programs. If you believe, as we do, that the benefits are worth taking a few precautionary measures for, then you are ready to get started. We suggest you begin by selecting footwear and attire that are appropriate for you and your active lifestyle. In addition, you will want to begin monitoring your resting heart rate. This chapter will help you through these endeavors.

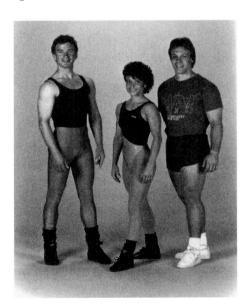

SELECTING APPROPRIATE ATTIRE

Selecting the proper attire for a creative aerobic fitness class is important and relatively easy if you observe a few basic guidelines. Generally, you should choose clothes that are suitable for the exercise environment, and those that are made from cotton or cotton based fabric. In cold weather, layers of clothing are recommended. As your body temperature rises and the muscles are warmed you can take off what you do not need. In warm weather, clothing made from cotton is desirable. Cotton fabric allows your body to maintain its normal temperature by pulling perspiration away from the skin. As clothing becomes damp, the surrounding air causes the moisture to evaporate and enables the body to cool and perspire freely. Nylon and polyester fabrics, while fashionable, are not recommended because they do not absorb perspiration or allow body heat to escape. This may result in an undesirable rise in body temperature, an increase in water loss and fatigue. Body wraps made of rubber and plastic are actually dangerous because the heat retention is intensified and serious dehydration may occur. Any reduction in weight is due to water loss not lower body fat. Drinking liquids of any kind will quickly rehydrate the tissues, returning the body to its original weight.

Aerobic enthusiasts are encouraged to purchase cotton leotards, tights, shirts, shorts or sweat suits. Athletic bras should be worn by women and athletic supports should be worn by men to reduce strain caused by jarring.

SELECTING A PERFORMANCE SHOE

Selecting the proper footwear for a creative aerobic fitness class is essential in terms of injury prevention. Athletic shoes are designed to minimize injury and enhance performance. Most athletic shoes are sport specific. That is, the foot movements executed during one activity are not the same as the movements performed in another. During running, for example, the foot lands heel to toe, while in aerobic dance the general foot pattern is toe to heel and back to the toe. As a result, running shoes are not appropriate for an aerobic dance class. Cross-training shoes, however, are designed for a variety of activities and can be used very effectively for aerobic dance, stepping, sliding, and jumping rope.

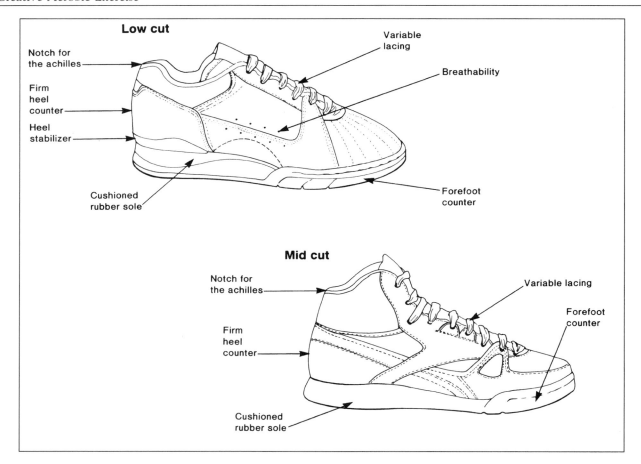

Low cut

Notch for
the achilles

Firm
heel
counter

Heel
stabilizer

Cushioned
rubber sole

Variable
lacing

Breathability

Forefoot
counter

Mid cut

Notch for
the achilles

Firm
heel
counter

Cushioned
rubber sole

Variable lacing

Forefoot
counter

Figure 1

In general, a good aerobic shoe is light weight, flexible, built to absorb shock and reinforced to prevent unnecessary heel movement. The shoe exterior should be made of soft leather and capable of bending without a lot of resistance. If a shoe does not bend easily, it will be too stiff and possibly uncomfortable during the aerobic workout. Good aerobic shoes have a well cushioned inner sole with a substantial amount of cushioning in the forefoot. They also have a soft midsole under both the forefoot and heel which adds extra cushioning for running and jumping movements on hard surfaces.

Participating in aerobic dance will take your life in many new directions . . . literally. You'll move forward, backwards, to the side, and even in circles, but not necessarily in that order. Because of the dynamic and creative movements in aerobic dance your shoes need to be supportive, especially when turning or moving to the side. Shoes that are reinforced between the upper sole and the forefoot and have a stiff heel counter will help prevent unnecessary inward or outward movement of the foot.

When shopping for shoes, choose a store that specializes in athletic shoes. It may also help if you tell the salesperson the type of floor surface you will be exercising on and the type of foot you have (high arch, low arch, no arch, pain or previous injury). Hard surfaces, such as concrete or wood, require shoes that have more cushion in the toe, arch and heel to help absorb the force of jumping and running. Floor surfaces that are cushioned, such as mats, carpeting, or spring floors, need less cushioning but require a smooth outer sole on the shoe to allow for easy side to side movements.

Check your feet to see if they pronate, supinate or are normal. **Pronation** means that your *foot rolls inward, causing the arch of the foot to flatten* (Figure 2). A heavy pronator often lacks the muscular support necessary to maintain a neutral or normal foot pattern. As a result, the muscles that support the arch must work harder. You should purchase a shoe that has a firm mid sole (arch region) and heel counter to keep the heel from moving medially in the shoe. **Supination** means that your *foot rolls outward, resulting in wear on the*

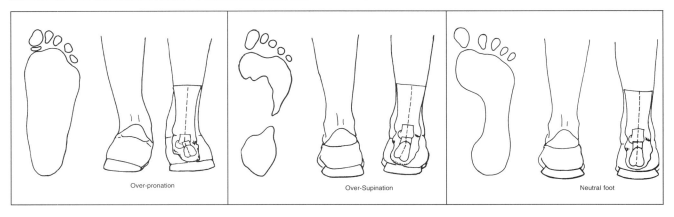

Figure 2   Figure 3   Figure 4

outside of the shoe (Figure 3). A heavy supinator often has a high arch and rigid foot. A supinator also needs a shoe that has extra support with a special emphasis on maintaining a neutral foot position.

Extra support is directly related to injury prevention. A normal foot pattern begins with the outer part of the heel striking the ground first in a slightly supinated position. As the foot moves forward the body weight shifts and rolls the foot inward flattening the arch (pronation). Pronation continues until the weight is transferred forward to the inside ball of the foot to the toe-off position. The combination of supination and pronation allows the foot to adapt to changing terrain.

Plan to spend some time in the store trying on and comparing several pairs of aerobic shoes. Test each pair by running, jumping or doing your favorite aerobic step. Check to see that the shoe fits snugly in all phases of movement, but not so tight that your toes feel cramped. Comfort is very important. Be sure the shoes you buy feel good.

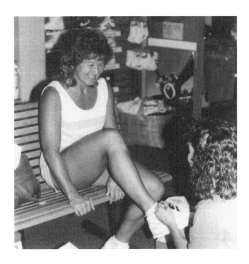

Replacing Worn Shoes

Any shoe worn regularly will experience wear. Because of the demand placed on athletic shoes, you can expect to replace them, but when? The most vulnerable part of an aerobic shoe is the cushioning. Because the material is soft, it will eventually compress and fail to absorb shock. As you will find out in more detail in chapter 12, replacing worn shoes is an important factor in injury prevention. Yet, you can't judge ongoing performance by appearance alone. Like selecting the right shoe in the first place, you must put the shoes on and feel the effects. When evaluating your shoes for wear realize that discomfort in your feet, shins, knees, or back could be related to your shoes.

A shoe worn regularly for indoor exercise (not for leisure or wearing around campus) will last anywhere from three to six months. Other factors

---

TABLE 3-1
Can Your Aerobic Shoes Pass This Test?

Ask yourself, are your shoes:

- flexible, bending easily at the forefoot without much resistance?
- supportive, stabilizing the foot through movement in all directions?
- cushioned, absorbing shock and minimizing landing forces?
- less than 3–6 months old (if worn regularly)?

If you said NO to any of the above questions, you may be setting yourself up for an unnecessary injury. Remember, worn shoes need to be replaced.

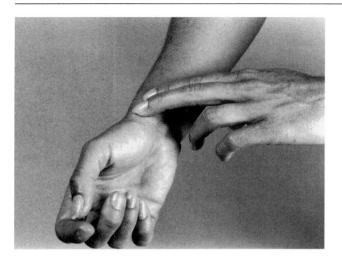

Radial Pulse

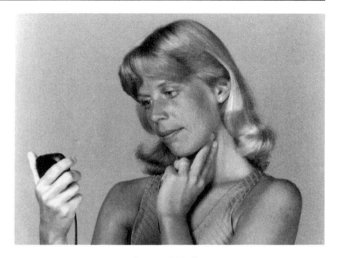

Carotid Pulse

related to shoe wear is the body weight of the participant and the impact level of the activity being performed. High impact activities and greater body weight will break down a shoe more quickly. If you already have a pair of athletic shoes, please take these guidelines into consideration before you use "any old shoes" for another aerobic dance class.

THE RESTING HEART RATE

The heart rate response to exercise is considered the single best indicator of cardiovascular fitness. Heart rate is easy to measure and is used to monitor various activities. You can find your pulse by using either the radial or carotid artery. To locate the radial artery, place the tips of your index and middle finger of your right hand on the left wrist in the small groove below the base of your left thumb. To locate the carotid artery, place the tips of the same two fingers on the same side of your neck, under the jaw bone, about midway between the chin and the ear. Hold your fingertips on one of these points with sufficient pressure to feel the artery pulsating. Each pulsation reflects a heart beat. Count the number of beats felt during one full minute.

The resting heart rate should be taken at a time when the body is truly at rest. The best time is just after waking while still lying in bed, assuming that you have not been startled awake by your alarm clock. To get the most representative value, the resting heart rate should be measured and recorded over a five day period and then averaged.

Resting heart rates vary among individuals and are directly related to cardiovascular fitness. Highly

conditioned long distance runners, for example, often have resting heart rates between 30 and 40 beats per minute, while sedentary individuals typically demonstrate values above 80 beats per minute. Ideally, the lower the heart rate, the less work the heart has to do as more blood enters the heart chamber between beats. Thus, the body receives a larger volume of oxygenated blood and nutrients. Moderately physically active individuals will generally have resting heart rates between 60 and 80 beats per minute. As a person continues to become more aerobically conditioned, the evidence will be reflected in a lowered resting heart rate.

University students enrolled in creative aerobic fitness classes may want to monitor their resting heat rate (Apppendix A).

SUMMARY

Selecting the appropriate attire and footwear for a class in creative aerobic fitness is the first step to insuring an injury free experience. Cotton attire that allows freedom of movement is highly recommended. An aerobic shoe that provides forefoot flexibility, shock absorption, lateral stability, a good fit, comfort and extra support unique to your foot pattern is important. The next step is to monitor your resting heart rate and calculate an accurate average. This information can then be used to determine your individual training heart rate which will serve as an indicator of aerobic intensity. Having completed these initial steps, you are well prepared to begin the exercise portion of your class. Smile, take a big breath and get ready.

GLOSSARY

Neutral Position (of the foot and ankle)—a position that is neither supinated nor pronated and one that minimizes stress to the ankle, foot and lower extremity.

Pronation (of the foot and ankle)—inward rotation of the ankle joint that causes the arch of the foot to flatten.

Resting Heart Rate—a measure and indicator of heart function when the body is lying still. Most often monitored just upon waking.

Supination (of the foot and ankle)—outward rotation of the ankle joint that places additional weight on the outer soles of the feet.

REFERENCES

Dufek, J. S. & Bates, B. T. (1991). Dynamic performance assessment of selected sport shoes on impact forces. *Medicine and Science in Sports and Exercise, 23* (9), 1062–1067.

Nigg, B. M. & Segesser, B. (1992). Biomechanical and orthopedic concepts in sport shoe construction. *Medicine and Science in Sports and Exercise, 24* (5), 595–602.

PART II

PROGRAM DEVELOPMENT

The challenges of change are always hard . . . realize that we each have a role that requires us to change and become more responsible for shaping our own future.

–Hillary Rodham Clinton

CHAPTER 4

The Building Blocks for a Total Program

Although aerobic exercise is the most important component of a creative fitness program, it is not the only one. In fact, one of the advantages of choosing a creative aerobic fitness program over, or in conjunction with other aerobic exercise such as jogging or cycling, is that it provides a means for enhancing motor ability and, more importantly, for achieving *total fitness*.

PHYSICAL FITNESS AND MOTOR ABILITY

Physical fitness is most often defined as *the ability to carry out daily tasks and strenuous physical activities with vigor and without excessive fatigue*. Physical fitness is directly related to *health*. Fit individuals are more likely to lead healthy and productive lives, with less risk of coronary heart disease, obesity and lower back problems, than are unfit individuals.

Motor ability, on the other hand, *is related to skill or skillful performance of an activity*. The components of motor ability include speed, power, reaction time, agility, coordination, balance and rhythm or timing. Undoubtedly you remember picking teams in physical education classes. There were the natural athletes that everyone wanted on their team and then there were those who were selected last. These selections were most often a reflection of innate motor ability. Fortunately, creative aerobic fitness programs are designed for everyone, regardless of motor ability. They are non-competitive and allow for individual expression and interpretation of the instructor's movements. It really doesn't matter if you can change directions quickly, stay with the beat, or coordinate your arms and legs as well as your instructor because the primary goal of these programs is to enhance aerobic fitness, not motor ability. However, research does demonstrate that individual motor ability will improve with practice. Thus, regular participation in a creative aerobic fitness program is certain to enhance your motor skills as you strive to attain and maintain the benefits of health-related fitness.

HEALTH-RELATED PHYSICAL FITNESS

Health-related physical fitness is concerned with preventing coronary heart disease, low back pain, problems associated with being overweight, muscle and joint disorders, and the physiological complications attributed to stress. The five components of health-related physical fitness essential for leading a healthy life are <u>flexibility</u>, <u>cardiorespiratory endurance</u>, <u>body composition</u>, <u>muscular strength</u> and <u>muscular endurance</u>. These same components serve as the building blocks for a total creative aerobic fitness program.

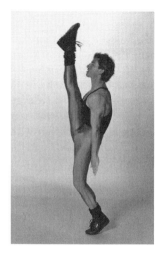

Flexibility

Flexibility is defined as *the range of motion at a joint and its corresponding muscle groups*. The ability to move each joint in the body through its full range of motion enhances movement efficiency, decreases muscle soreness, and lessens the possibility of injury to muscles, tendons, ligaments and joints. Good flexibility may help prevent low back pain, which can be attributed, in part, to tightness of the muscles located in the back of the thighs, hips and lower back. To evaluate your flexibility refer to the assessments described in the next chapter.

Once you have assessed your flexibility you can improve your range of motion by engaging in a series of slow, static stretches for all of the major joints and/or muscle groups in the body. It is important not to stretch, however, until the muscles in the body have been warmed-up sufficiently. Chapter 6 describes how to stretch safely and effectively during a typical workout.

Cardiorespiratory Endurance (Aerobic Endurance)

Cardiorespiratory endurance, *the primary component and single best measure of health-related physical fitness is concerned with the body's ability to deliver oxygen to the muscles and all of its vital organs during sustained exercise*. It involves two life supporting systems in the body, namely the cardiovascular system (heart and blood vessels) and the respiratory system (lungs).

Your heart is the most important muscle in your body. It beats an average of 100,000 times per day at rest pumping nearly 2,000 gallons of oxygenated blood through the circulatory system. It beats continuously, keeping you alive. If you want it to become stronger and stay healthy it must be exercised like any other muscle in the body. When exercised regularly its strength increases. When it is not exercised, its strength decreases. When it stops, you stop. Preventing coronary heart disease or reducing the risk of a subsequent heart attack requires proper conditioning and good nutritional care.

Your lungs work in conjunction with the heart to supply every cell in your body with an adequate and continuous supply of oxygen. Oxygen, attached to the hemoglobin molecule, is carried in the bloodstream to provide energy for cell metabolism. Carbon dioxide is the waste product. The gases diffuse through two very thin cell layers that separate air in the alveoli (tiny sacs in the lung walls)

from the blood in the capillaries. When insufficient oxygen is delivered to the muscles, their ability to function is reduced. Rapid and shallow breathing, typical of a sedentary person, puts a strain on the heart that results in an increase in heart rate and blood pressure.

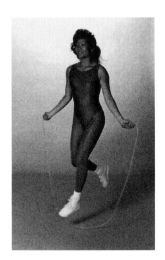

The more active you are, the more oxygen you need. How hard your cardiorespiratory system must work depends on the level of cardiorespiratory endurance you have and how efficient your muscles are at using oxygen during aerobic exercise. You can evaluate your present aerobic endurance by using one of the assessments described in Chapter 5. Following the fitness guidelines found in Chapter 7 and the program ideas described in Chapter 8, you will learn how you can improve your cardiorespiratory endurance.

Body Composition

Body composition *refers to that portion of the body that consists of fat (adipose tissue) as opposed to lean tissue (bones, muscles, and internal organs)*. The percentage of fat in one's body is a more accurate indicator of fitness and health than body weight as depicted on height-weight charts. Excess fat is not healthy due to the extra weight and stress that it places on your heart. Too little fat is not healthy either because the body relies on it for energy, insulation, protection and storage of the fat soluble vitamins A, D, E and K. Generally, women have a higher percentage of body fat than men due to an extra layer of fat below the skin. This additional layer serves as the primary site for the conversion of androgens to estrogens, essential for menstruation and reproduction. While there is some disagreement as to the "optimal" range of body fat, a roundtable of experts did recommend that women maintain their body fat between 16–25% and men between 12–18% (Wilmore, 1986). However, even with training both bone density and lean tissue tend to decrease with age. As a result, a few percentage points can be added for both older men and women.

Recommended percentages do not necessarily represent the ideal for all individuals. But they do serve as a guide and are generally accepted. It is not uncommon, however, to find a much lower percentage of body fat in healthy people who participate regularly in aerobic or endurance type activities. Long distance runners for example, typically measure between 5%–10% for men and 10%–15% for women. Dedicated sports enthusiasts often take on body characteristics specific to their sport, creating a lean to fat ratio that maximizes energy and increases efficiency during performance.

Muscular individuals may appear overweight according to height-weight charts, yet many possess very little body fat. This is because muscle weighs almost twice as much as fat. It makes sense, therefore, to use the term "overfat" rather than "overweight" when discussing weight management. This might be a good time to persuade those of you who weigh yourselves on the bathroom scale to think about an alternative. If you are gaining muscle weight through exercise the scale will show an increase in total body weight. This increase can be psychologically defeating and serve no real purpose. It would make more sense to have your body composition measured periodically to assess the effects of your exercise program. Throw the bathroom scale away! It only measures daily fluctuations in total body weight and provides no information concerning the fat and lean make-up of your body. Methods for determining your body composition are described in Chapter 5. Details on nutrition, diet and exercise are reserved for Chapters 11 and 12.

Muscular Strength and Endurance

Muscular strength *refers to the amount of force you can produce with a single maximal effort against a resistance while lifting, moving or pushing.* **Muscular endurance** *is a sub-maximal force that occurs repeatedly or a sustained contraction that is held for a period of time.* Optimal levels of strength and muscular endurance vary with different activities, but minimal levels are needed to prevent injury. Strong abdominal muscles are essential for good health because they form a solid support for your internal

organs and prevent the back from hyperextending—another cause of lower back pain.

The best way to build strength and/or muscular endurance is through a structured and supervised weight lifting program. In general, strength is developed with heavy weights and few repetitions. Muscular endurance is developed with lighter weights and more repetitions. For achieving total fitness, weight training programs or progressive resistance exercises are often recommended in addition to aerobic exercise programs.

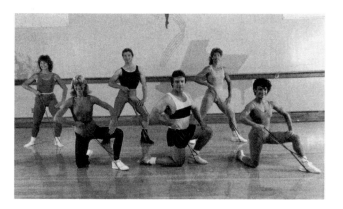

Creative aerobic fitness programs, with their emphasis on total conditioning, build as much abdominal, upper body and lower body work into their programs as possible. The use of light weights and elastic bands, as well as, specific exercise suggestions are described in Chapter 9. To familiarize yourself with the major muscle groups study figure 4-1.

POSTURE

"Sit up straight! Stop slouching!" Sound familiar? How often did you hear those words as you were growing up? It may have seemed like too many at the time, but your friends and family were only trying to help. Chances are good that the postural habits you developed either affect your life today or have the potential to do so. Incorrect or poor posture can lead to back, neck and lower extremity injury and to a lifetime of unnecessary pain. This section will describe the elements of good and bad posture as they relate to exercise.

When an individual assumes correct posture there is a balanced relationship between the postural muscles and minimal strain on the muscles, tendons and ligaments of the weight bearing joints

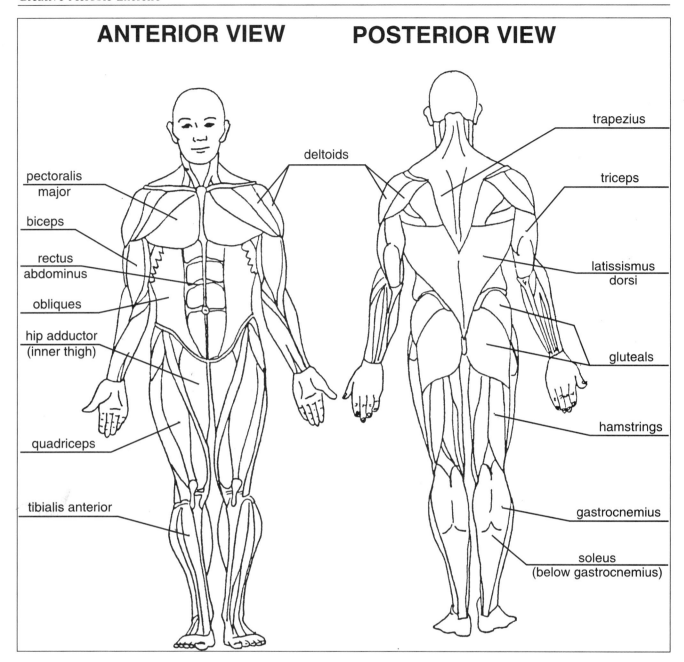

ANTERIOR VIEW

pectoralis
major

biceps

rectus
abdominus

obliques

hip adductor
(inner thigh)

quadriceps

tibialis anterior

deltoids

POSTERIOR VIEW

trapezius

triceps

latissismus
dorsi

gluteals

hamstrings

gastrocnemius

soleus
(below gastrocnemius)

Figure 4-1

of the body (Figure 4-2). Postural muscles are located on the anterior (front) and posterior (back) sides of the body. These muscles play an important role in helping the skeletal framework resist the force of gravity. Normally the body segments are balanced in a vertical column. If the postural muscles are not conditioned to resist the pull of gravity, one or more segments will move out of alignment. If any part of the body is out of line, the weight distribution becomes uneven, putting stress on the muscles and the musculoskeletal system.

Well conditioned postural muscles help to maintain the normal alignment of the spinal column with its three distinct curves: cervical (neck region) thoracic (upper/mid-back) and lumbar (low back) (Figure 4-3). These curves maintain an equal distribution of weight through all the segments of the spine. During movement these curves support the body, adapting to internal and external changes, including the pull of gravity. If the muscles on one side of the spine are stronger than those of the opposing side, the spine is pulled in the direction

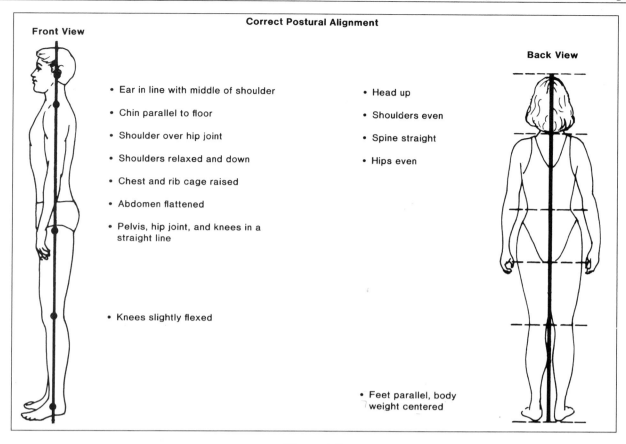

Correct Postural Alignment

Front View

- Ear in line with middle of shoulder
- Chin parallel to floor
- Shoulder over hip joint
- Shoulders relaxed and down
- Chest and rib cage raised
- Abdomen flattened
- Pelvis, hip joint, and knees in a straight line
- Knees slightly flexed

Back View

- Head up
- Shoulders even
- Spine straight
- Hips even

- Feet parallel, body weight centered

Figure 4-2

of the stronger muscles, increasing stress and pressure on the weaker side. When an individual carries excess weight across the abdomen, the muscles become stretched and weak, while the muscles of the lower back shorten. To correct this misalignment, the individual needs to strengthen the abdominal muscles and stretch the lower back muscles, gluteals and hamstrings (Figure 4-3).

As no two bodies are identical, no two people have the same posture concerns. You can correct or maintain your posture through proper conditioning, stretching, strengthening and care of the muscles and ligaments that determine postural alignment, thus ensuring better, if not "perfect" posture.

BREATHING DURING EXERCISE

Have you ever had trouble catching your breath? Maybe this happened after running up a flight of stairs or hiking in the mountains? The experience of breathlessness can be uncomfortable and even frightening. This sensation is your body's way of telling you that you're doing too much. Quite sim-

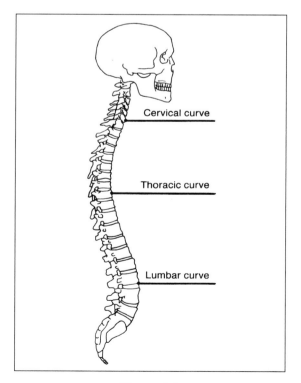

Cervical curve

Thoracic curve

Lumbar curve

Figure 4-3

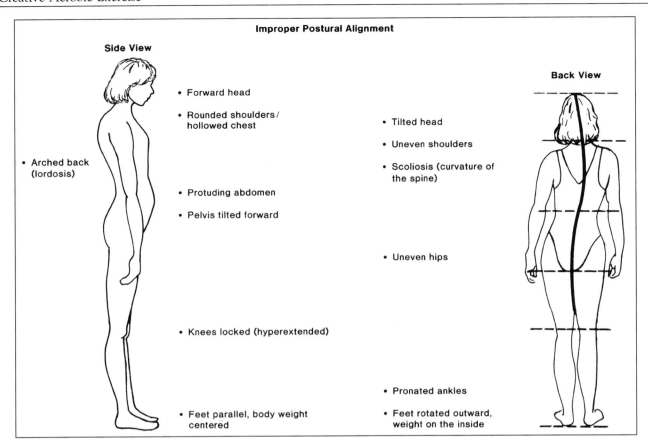

Improper Postural Alignment

Side View

- Forward head
- Rounded shoulders / hollowed chest
- Arched back (lordosis)
- Protuding abdomen
- Pelvis tilted forward
- Knees locked (hyperextended)
- Feet parallel, body weight centered

Back View

- Tilted head
- Uneven shoulders
- Scoliosis (curvature of the spine)
- Uneven hips
- Pronated ankles
- Feet rotated outward, weight on the inside

Figure 4-4

ply, your heart is unable to deliver enough oxygen to your muscles. Remembering that physical fitness is the ability to accomplish challenging physical activity without fatigue or discomfort, you can see that becoming breathless during exercise is not necessary. To minimize the "out of breath" feeling you need to maintain a moderate intensity, breathe deeply, and avoid holding your breath during activity.

A conscious effort should be made to continue steady state rhythmical breathing (through mouth and nose) during all aspects of the aerobic program. Holding your breath simply reduces the blood and oxygen flow to the brain and working muscles. As a result, fatigue can set in making the exercise labored and difficult. Breath holding occurs most often during the muscular endurance segment and seems to be an automatic response during a difficult exercise. Students should concentrate on inhalation during the recovery phase and exhalation during the work phase of each exercise. Adjust the pace of your activity to insure proper breathing mechanics.

SUMMARY

Creative aerobic fitness programs provide the ways and means to enhanced motor ability, health related physical fitness and posture. In the course of 8–12 weeks, diligent exercisers will begin to see improvement in agility, coordination, rhythm, flexibility, strength, muscular endurance, cardiorespiratory endurance, body composition and body alignment. Naturally, those who continue beyond the 12 weeks will continue to improve and reap the benefits that are rightfully theirs.

GLOSSARY

Body Composition—the percentage of fat to non-fat tissue in relation to total body weight.

Cardiorespiratory Endurance—the ability of the circulatory and respiratory systems to supply a continuous flow of oxygen to the muscles during sustained exercise.

Flexibility—the range of motion available in a joint.

Motor Ability—related to skill or skillful performance of an activity.

Muscular Endurance—a sub-maximal force produced with repeated contractions or a sustained contraction against a resistance.

Muscular Strength—the amount of force produced with a single maximal effort against a resistance while lifting, moving or pushing.

Physical Fitness—the ability to carry out daily tasks and strenuous activities with vigor and without excessive fatigue. The fact that physical fitness is related to health minimizes the risk of developing hypokinetic disease (disorders that limit one's ability for movement of the muscular, skeletal or cardiorespiratory systems).

REFERENCES

Casperson, C. J., Powell, K. E., & Christenson, G. M. (1985). Physical activity, exercise, and physical fitness: Definition and distinction for health-related research. *Public Health Reports, 100* (2), 126–131.

Wilmore, J. H. (1986). Body composition: A roundtable. *The Physician and Sportsmedicine, 14* (3), 144–162.

Obstacles often are not personal attacks; they are muscle builders
—Anne Wilson Schaef

CHAPTER 5

Tests and Measurements

So you want to start an exercise program. Where do you begin? The best way to initiate a safe and effective exercise program is to assess your present level of conditioning. The results of tests and measurements can be prescriptive as well as motivational. The results also serve as a baseline or starting point so that you can observe your progress. In the previous chapter we discussed the components for health related fitness. Using specific tests to assess these components we can evaluate one aspect of fitness or your total physical condition. Assessment, in conjunction with a personal health history and list of activity preferences, is helpful in designing and prescribing an individualized exercise program.

The purpose of this chapter is to highlight some of the techniques used to assess aerobic fitness, flexibility, muscular strength and endurance, and body composition both in a controlled laboratory setting and in the field. Advantages and disadvantages of each assessment will be presented and should serve as a guide when selecting tests and measurements appropriate to your needs.

EXERCISE TESTING

Exercise testing, which measures physiological function, varies from the sophisticated laboratory set-up to a simple field test. The use of the more precise laboratory tests versus a field test depends on the facility and equipment available, the size of the group being evaluated, and the time allotted for assessment. Both approaches can be used to help students identify their present fitness level, establish goals, and provide motivation. The results of any physical test, however, are relative and may not be absolutely precise. There can even be significant differences between the results of two laboratory tests designed to evaluate the same component of fitness. Evaluating body composition

using underwater weighing or skinfold measurements may yield different levels of body fat. Additional variability may occur when comparing individual results to the reference models that serve as standards. At best any physical assessment may only be a reliable estimate. Nevertheless, the results of a physical assessment can provide a baseline measure of general physical function and work capacity. Using the same testing procedures to compare an initial assessment or pre-test with a post evaluation (taken after a period of training), will provide the most useful means for monitoring progress.

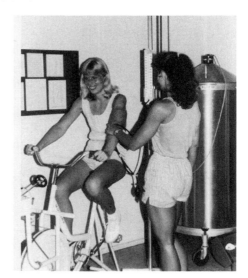

LABORATORY TESTING

Laboratory testing generally requires equipment and specific procedures. However, the primary difference between field tests and laboratory procedures is not fancy equipment, but the training and expertise of individuals administering the evaluation. Some procedures may even require several trained persons to perform the test. The laboratory procedures commonly used to evaluate cardiovascular capacity, muscular function, range of motion, and body composition will be outlined here.

Evaluating Cardiovascular Function

The laboratory tests that evaluate cardiovascular function are designed to measure aerobic capacity. **Aerobic capacity** *describes how the cardiorespiratory system responds to the increasing demands of a given activity and is evaluated by measuring one's ability to take in and utilize oxygen.*

A laboratory graded exercise test or "stress test" is typically administered on a treadmill or stationary bicycle ergometer. The exercise may be performed at either a *maximal* or *sub-maximal* effort. While the sub-max test is most common, the max-test is usually reserved as a diagnostic measure when there is a specific medical concern. The individual can usually request either test. During a maximal test, blood pressure is monitored and an electrocardiograph tracks the electrical activity of the heart. A participant begins with a brief warm-up on a treadmill or bicycle ergometer followed by an exercise session. The participant continues until the point of exhaustion. This method has been shown to be quite valuable in identifying cardiorespiratory pathologies at very high levels of physical activity.

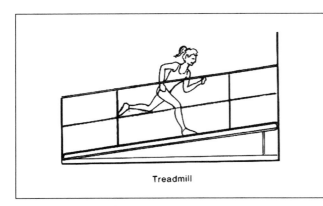

Treadmill

A sub-max test also begins with a brief warm-up period but is followed by an exercise period not lasting more than twelve minutes. The participant will be asked to walk or run on a level treadmill or pedal at a low resistance on the bicycle ergometer at a given speed. Speed of the activity is dictated by the type of exercise and established guidelines or test protocol. When the heart rate reaches a predetermined submaximal level, such as 75% of maximum, the test is terminated. Aerobic capacity is then indirectly determined from the heart rate

and mechanical workload. The results are compared with norms and an exercise prescription is given.

Choosing between the treadmill or bicycle ergometer modes of testing will depend on whether your activities involve cycling or walking/running. We recommended that you select the mode which best simulates the activity you are currently involved in, or about to begin.

Evaluating Body Composition

There are several methods used to assess the relative percentages of fat and non-fat (lean) tissue. These include hydrostatic (underwater) weighing and skinfold measures. The hydrostatic weighing and skinfold methods provide good estimations of body composition when the tests are conducted properly. Values obtained from the two methods may differ somewhat, but each provides a baseline from which to compare results from subsequent assessments.

Hydrostatic weighing is considered the most accurate of all methods used to evaluate body composition and is available at many colleges and most universities at a reasonable cost. Comparisons are made between an individual's dry land weight and their weight in water. Body composition when measured by a trained professional is rather simple, involving the total emersion of a person in a tank of warm water. The scale attached to the special chair in the tank records your underwater weight. To make this test more accurate a measurement of lung volume should be taken. This will account for air in the lungs during submersion. Through a series of complex computations fat and non-fat

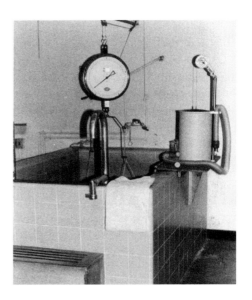

tissue percentages are derived. All other assessment techniques are compared to hydrostatic weighing.

Although not as accurate, the skinfold method of evaluating body composition is often used in the laboratory, as well as in the field setting. This method involves the use of calipers which measure skinfolds at various sites on the body. Measures are recorded and computed in a formula which provides an estimated ratio of fat to non-fat tissue. Unfortunately, there are so many formulas to choose from that the results may vary considerably. Some formulas call for as many as ten skinfold sites while others only measure two sites. Most fitness experts agree that the sum of several sites provides the most representative assessment of body composition. Regardless of the formula selected, if the same method is accurately repeated during reassessment, changes in body composition will be evident.

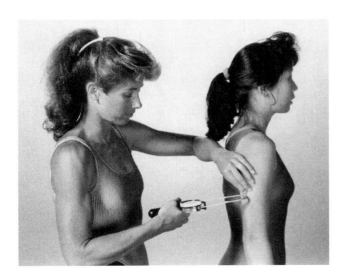

Evaluating Muscular Function

As described in the previous chapter there is a definite distinction between muscular strength and endurance, the difference being the intensity and the duration of the effort. In evaluating strength and endurance, an additional distinction is made between dynamic and static effort. Static describes the tension developed in the muscle without movement, while dynamic refers to the muscular effort during movement. Dynamometers are devices that can measure both static strength and/or endurance. To evaluate static strength, the subject exerts maximal force by pushing or pulling and then records the pressure. To evaluate endurance, muscle contraction is maintained for 60 seconds and tension is recorded in 10 second intervals. The two most

common dynamometers evaluate hand grip and low back/leg strength.

Dynamic strength and endurance can also be evaluated by specialized isokinetic machines. These machines assess muscle strength by controlling the range of motion and speed of the movement. These machines don't have to be set at a specific weight like conventional weight machines but are able to accommodate the amount of resistance applied by the contracting muscle. This makes the machines safe to use for observing maximum effort without concern of over-exertion or injury.

Evaluating Flexibility

Precise measurements of range of motion are evaluated with an instrument called a goniometer. This "protractor-like device" provides a direct measure of joint angle. After placing the apex on any joint, a rotating arm measures the number of degrees of movement in the corresponding limb. This instrument is often used by physical therapists and is an important tool in rehabilitation as injuries may limit range of motion in a joint. By using the goniometer, a therapist can monitor progress while re-establishing normal range of motion.

FIELD TESTING

Field testing has been designed as an alternate method to assess various components of physical fitness when a laboratory is not accessible. Field tests work well with large groups, do not require trained professionals, and can be performed in a minimal amount of time. Many of these tests allow the participant to evaluate himself/herself or a partner, thus teaching them about evaluation and assessment. While lack of formal training may make these tests less than 100% accurate or reliable, the results provide excellent baseline measures. When a baseline assessment is followed by additional measurements using the same initial method, progress can be effectively monitored.

Evaluating Aerobic Fitness

Aerobic fitness can be evaluated using stepping, walking or jogging. There are simple fitness tests that can be safely administered to a variety of participants, with minimal equipment in a short amount of time. Using a stop watch, a metronome (or pre-recorded tape), and a twelve inch platform, a step test can be used to evaluate the recovery heart rate after three minutes of exercise. This test evaluates aerobic capacity by assessing how quickly the heart recovers from a structured activity. Each participant steps up and down on the platform at an established cadence. After stepping the participant immediately sits down and monitors the post-activity pulse. A more fit individual will not work as hard while stepping and will recover more quickly from exercise, resulting in a lower post-activity heart rate. Procedures for the test and results can be found in table 5-1.

If step platforms are not available, a one-mile walk or a mile-and-half walk/jog can be used just as effectively. The only equipment required is a stop watch, pencil, paper and a predetermined course. A track is a convenient site for this test but any other flat, measured area will suffice. The goal is to cover the appropriate distance as fast as possible. The

---

TABLE 5-1
3-Minute Step Test for Measuring Aerobic Endurance

For this activity you will need a watch and a 12-inch-high step.

Directions

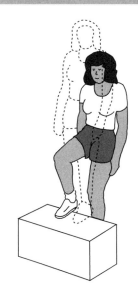

1. Before warming-up take a one minute pre-activity heart rate.

2. Complete a brief warm-up (1–2 minutes) and be sure to stretch legs.

3. For 3 minutes, step up and down on the step in a four-part movement: (a) up with the left foot, (b) up with the right foot, (c) down with the left foot, (d) down with the right foot.

4. You can alternate your lead foot, but try to keep pace at 24 steps a minute. (Each step is a four-part movement.)

5. Immediately after the 3 minutes, sit down and check your pulse for one minute.

6. Compare your results to the table below.

Women	Step test—Recovery heart rate				
Age	Excellent	High	Average	Low	Very Low
Under 30	72–84	85–108	109–116	117–135	136–155
30–39	74–86	87–107	108–117	118–136	137–154
40–49	74–90	91–112	113–118	119–131	132–152
50–59	76–92	93–112	113–120	121–134	135–152
60 and older	74–90	91–109	110–119	120–133	134–151

Men	Step test—Recovery heart rate				
Age	Excellent	High	Average	Low	Very Low
Under 30	70–78	79–97	98–105	106–126	127–164
30–39	72–80	81–100	101–109	110–126	127–168
40–49	74–82	83–103	104–113	114–128	129–168
50–59	72–84	85–104	105–115	116–130	131–154
60 and older	72–86	87–101	102–110	111–128	129–150

Source: The President's Council on Physical Fitness, YMCA.
Adapted from Williams, B. K. & Knight, S. M. (1993). *Healthy for life: Wellness and the art of living.* Pacific Grove, CA: Brooks/ Cole Publishing.

difference in distance relates back to the necessary duration of a test designed to estimate aerobic capacity. Tests designed to evaluate aerobic conditioning should last between 9–12 minutes. A one mile run or even walk/jog can be completed by trained individuals in as little as six minutes. On the other hand, completing a mile and a half walk may take many people more than twelve minutes and result in fatigue to the leg muscles rather than to the cardiovascular system.

Experienced runners or individuals with an established aerobic program can run or combine running with walking for a mile and a half. Inexperienced runners or apparently healthy individuals just starting an exercise program can use the one mile walk format. This is a safer option for anyone not physically trained for jogging. All participants should warm-up prior to starting and be sure to carefully cool down and stretch after the test. If using an outside facility, heat and humidity are also a performance factor. As these tests are designed to estimate aerobic capacity, care should be given to make sure the testing environment is conducive to maximal effort. Avoiding the heat and high humidity will increase performance. The results of these tests can be compared to table 5-2.

Evaluating Muscular Function

Muscular function can be evaluated using common calisthenic exercises including push-ups, curl-ups, and pull-ups. Whether these are actually measures of strength or endurance depends upon individual performance. Many individuals may only be able to do one pull-up or push-up. In that case these exercises would evaluate upper body strength. However, participants who can complete several dozen curl-ups would be assessing muscular endurance. Because of the variance in normative values, these tests work best when used as pre and post-tests. See table 5-4 for details on performing the test.

Evaluating Flexibility

Evaluating range of motion helps establish the presence of any muscle imbalances. When assessing individual muscles, it is not unusual to find that one leg or shoulder is tighter or less flexible than the other. This type of imbalance is not desirable and indicates areas that need to be targeted during flexibility training. Using the criteria set up in table 5-3, individuals can estimate their own flexibility. These tests can be performed using partners and if

more precise results are desired, a measuring tape can be used to measure the distance between actual and criterion values.

TABLE 5-2
One and a Half Mile Run/Walk

Goal: To run 1.5 miles as quickly as you can.

Directions:
1. Warm up prior to the test.
2. This is a test of your maximum capacity, so be prepared for a challenge. Cover the distance as fast as possible without overexerting. Keep an even pace, running as long as you can and walking when necessary.
3. Record your time to the nearest second.
4. Cool down by walking first then stretching.
5. Compare your time to the table below.

	Men	Women
Excellent	<8:26	<10:52
Good	8:26–10:21	10:52–13:40
Average	10:22–12:17	13:41–16:28
Poor	12:18–14:14	16:29–19:16
Very Poor	>14:14	>19:16

One Mile Walk

Goal: To walk one mile as quickly as you can.

Directions:
1. Warm-up and stretch prior to test.
2. Walk one mile as quickly as you can using proper technique.
3. Record your time to the nearest second.
4. Cool down and stretch.
5. Compare your time to the table below.

	Men	Women
Superior	<11:07	<12:02
Above Average	11:07–12:31	12:02–13:05
Average	12:32–13:56	13:06–14:10
Below Average	13:57–15:20	14:11–15:14
Poor	>15:20	>15:14

Adapted from Robbins, G., Powers, D., & Burgess, S. (1994). *A wellness way of life.* Madison, WI: WCB Brown & Benchmark.

TABLE 5-3

Exercise & Target Area	Position	Criteria
Sit and reach evaluates back and hamstrings	 seated using hands	while seated with both legs extended and knees slightly bent, touch toes with finger tips
Leg Flexion evaluates individual hamstrings	 supine without hands *evaluate right and left leg*	while lying on the back, achieve 90° angle from the floor to the back of the extended leg (no assisting with the hands)
Hip Flexion evaluates individual hip flexor	 supine using hands *evaluate right and left leg*	while lying on the back, bring the thigh to the chest, keeping the calf and heel of the other leg on the ground
Knee Flexion evaluates individual quadriceps	 prone with shoulders down and knees together and using one hand *evaluate right and left leg*	while laying on the stomach, bring the heel to touch the back of the hip (avoid pulling the knee to the side)
Shoulder Flexion and Extension evaluates individual arms & shoulders	 one arm up palm in; the other arm back with palm out *evaluate right and left side*	while standing, touch finger tips *behind* the back

TABLE 5-4

Goal	Activity	Objective	Equipment	Organization
Measure muscular function of the upper body	Push-ups from the toes or the knees	Complete as many push-ups as possible in 30 seconds	Mat and stop watch	Partners monitor form and count repetitions
Measure muscular function of the upper body	Pull-ups or 90° flexed arm hang	Complete as many pull-ups as possible or hold flexed arm position as long as possible	Pull-up bar and stop watch	Partners spot, count pull-ups or time arm hang
Measure muscular function of the trunk	Crunches with knees bent and arms to the side	Complete as many crunches as possible or in one minute	Mat and stop watch	Partners monitor form and count repetitions

Evaluating Body Composition

As discussed earlier, skinfold measurements are often used to assess body composition in the field setting. The instructor can take the measurements or partners can be used to evaluate each other. While this can be a very effective assessment tool when used by experienced professionals, the results are not as precise nor reliable when used by untrained or inexperienced individuals.

Several devices are on the market that can also be used to evaluate body composition. Systems using ultra-sound, infra-red light, electrical impedance, and anthropometric measurements all claim to measure body fat. Research shows varying results between these systems and underwater weighing. Certainly, if available, these devices can be used as a relative measurement. Similar to comparing variations in body weight using the same bathroom scale, the results from one of these devices can show relative changes in body composition. However, a lack of research accuracy may make these measurements less than precise and comparisons to normative tables unreliable.

Waist to Hip Ratio

While not a measure of body composition, research has evaluated the relationship between girth measurements and the risk of heart disease. Observing the body type of those already at risk for heart disease, a relationship between hip and waist measurement has been identified. Both men and women who carry excess weight around the mid-drift have been associated with an increased risk for developing heart disease. Gender differences show that men and women at greater risk tend to distribute this fat differently, but that it generally concentrates between the waist and hips. Though this assessment doesn't specifically evaluate body composition, it is an informative field test that can be easily evaluated. See table 5-5 for procedures.

TABLE 5-5
Waist-to-Hip Ratio

Sample equation:

Male: 40-inch waist and 38-inch hips

$40 \div 38 = 1.05$

The ratio indicates that this person has an increased risk of developing cardiovascular disease.

Recommended Standard
Men: <1.0
Women: <.85

Waist-to-Hip Ratio Computation

Waist (inches): _____
Hip (inches) _____

_____ ÷ _____ = _____
waist   hips   ratio

Compare this value to the recommended standard shown above.

Adapted from Hoeger, W. W. K., & Hoeger, S. A. (1993). *Fitness and wellness* (2nd ed.). Englewood, CO: Morton Publishing.

Girth Measurements

Another method commonly used to evaluate physical changes is to measure the girth of various segments of the body. While this method really tells you nothing about the relative composition of fat to non-fat tissue, it will provide you with quantitative information regarding changes in size. A regular aerobic program which also incorporates muscular strength and endurance exercises can have a profound effect on reshaping the body. We recommend that you take measurements at the following sites:

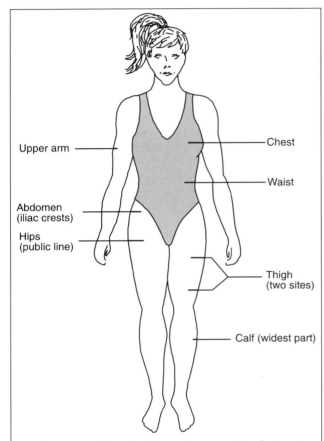

Upper arm

Abdomen (iliac crests)

Hips (public line)

Chest

Waist

Thigh (two sites)

Calf (widest part)

A suggested method to relocate original sites is to measure the distance from a near-by bony landmark to the measurement site and record the distance. Reassess every 3–6 months.

USING RESULTS TO ESTABLISH GOALS

Specialists in behavior and lifestyle development recognize the importance of identifying and establishing goals. **Goal setting** *is the first step to reinforcing an existing behavior or changing an unwanted habit.* Writing down intentions (objectives) and actions (outcomes) is one technique for monitoring the progress of your program and helping you achieve your goals. It is very important that your intentions and actions support your goals. Detailing individual workouts allows you and your instructor to compare your actions with the established guidelines for total fitness.

Goal Setting

The results of your fitness assessment provides you with information about your current level of fitness. With that information you can determine your fitness goals. Goal setting seems easy, but in order to establish effective goals you need to follow some specific guidelines. In developing and discussing your goals and objectives it is important to create ones that are *realistic* and *obtainable*. A goal should be specific, measurable, and designed to produce the desired results. Many personal goals are large endeavors that take time to achieve, especially in terms of exercise and diet. So as not to be overwhelmed and ultimately unsuccessful, be sure to establish several short-term goals that culminate to help you strive toward that larger, long-term goal. A short-term goal is a task that can be accomplished in one to four weeks. A long-term goal may take months or years to accomplish. Use short-term goals to evaluate your progress towards an ultimate goal.

Objectives

Objectives are the steps you use to achieve goals. If your long-term goal is to develop a regular fitness program, you need to identify how you plan to accomplish that. The first step is to choose a program that includes activities for flexibility, cardiovascular conditioning, muscular strength and muscular endurance. Then you must expand your objectives to state how many times a week you need exercise, what specific skills you will do and for how long. You might support these initial steps with additional objectives that will help reinforce your desired behavior. Recording your workouts on a log or calendar, using stairs rather than elevators, working out with an exercise partner are all objectives that support an active lifestyle.

Process and Product-Oriented Goals

In the discussion on motivation in chapter two, we established the importance of being involved in the process of exercise rather than just the products of activity. When developing your objectives consider the issues of ongoing motivation, select activities that you enjoy, and don't punish yourself with guilt for missing a workout. Just reschedule it. Product-oriented goals do not have to be avoided. Most of us desire accomplishments as a result of our endeavors and exercise is no different. However, in remembering what we have learned about motivation, it becomes important to support any product-oriented goals with additional goals that center upon the process of enjoying and participating in activity. Table 5-6 provides examples of product and process oriented fitness goals and the corresponding objectives.

SUMMARY

Evaluation of aerobic capacity, muscular strength/endurance, flexibility and body composition can provide you with a relatively good estimation of your current level of physical fitness. Results of such tests and measurements can also serve as a strong motivator to exercise. This holds true for the beginner, as well as for the long term exercise enthusiast. Each test method varies in degree of sophistication, cost, time and absolute accuracy. Regardless of the test you select, we suggest that you schedule periodic reassessments to evaluate your personal progress every 3–6 months.

Key Points to Remember

1. Select the exercise test that's appropriate to your needs.

2. Remember, each evaluation is an estimate and not an absolute value.

3. Use the initial assessment results as a baseline from which to make comparisons.

4. Beware! Do not compare the results of one test method to a different method, even if they are designed to measure the same variable, e.g., hydrostatic weighing compared to skinfold measurements will likely yield two different sets of numbers.

5. Only compare the results of identical tests and test methods.

6. Reassess between three and six months.

7. Be consistent with your exercise program if you want to see improvement.

TABLE 5-6

Process Oriented

Short-term Goal: To engage in regular (enjoyable) exercise/activity for four weeks

Objectives:
1. to climb the stairs at school rather than using the elevator
2. to sign up for dance lessons with a friend
3. to spend 15 minutes everyday stretching
4. to go on at least one day hike with friends

Long-term Goal: To maintain an active lifestyle by developing active habits

Objectives:
1. to sign up for a fitness class at school, recreation program or local club
2. to workout with a partner lifting weights 2–3× per week
3. increase moderate level aerobic conditioning to 3× per week, including two days of aerobics and one day of walking for 30 minutes.
4. to spend one Saturday a month hiking

Product Oriented

Short-term Goal: To lose 3 lbs in one month

Objectives:
1. to begin resistance training 2×/week, including push-ups and crunches
2. increase moderate level aerobic conditioning to 3× per week, including two days of aerobics and one day of walking for 30 minutes.
3. decrease dietary fat intake to 60 grams/day

Long-term Goal: To lose 8 lbs by the end of the semester

Objectives:
1. after six weeks increase cardiovascular conditioning to 4× week and add additional day of aerobic dance, step, or walking
2. maintain resistive training to 2× per week, adding exercises with dynabands and weights
3. maintain dietary fat intake between 40 and 60 grams/day

GLOSSARY

Girth Measurements—the circumference of body segments such as the chest, waist, arms, etc.

Laboratory vs. Field Testing—field testing is often used when fitness assessments are made with large groups of people and/or when sophisticated testing equipment is not available. Laboratory testing is individualized and takes more time, special equipment and trained personnel.

Long-term Goal—a large endeavor which will take six months or longer to accomplish.

Hydrostatic Weighing—refers to the method of weighing the body under water to measure body density, which is used to estimate proportions of lean body weight and body fat.

Recovery Heart Rate—the pulse count taken after the completion of an aerobic activity to ensure that the heart has returned to pre-activity levels.

Short-term Goal—an endeavor which can easily be accomplished in less than a month.

Skinfold Technique—a method used to measure subcutaneous skinfolds at various sites on the body to predict body density and the relative proportions of lean body weight to body fat.

Waist-to-hip Ratio—an assessment comparing the measurements of the waist and hip in order to evaluate an individual's risk of heart disease.

REFERENCES

Baranowski, T., Bouchard, C., Bar-Or, O., Bricker, T., Heath, G., Kimm, S. Y. S., Malina, R., Obarzanek, E., Pate, R., Strong, W. B., Truman, B. & Washington, R. (1992). Assessment, prevalence and cardiovascular benefits of physical activity in youth. *Medicine and Science in Sports and Exercise, 24* (6), Supplement, S237–S245.

Corbin, C. B. & Lindsey, R. (1994). *Concepts of physical fitness with laboratories* (8th ed.). Dubuque, IA: Wm C. Brown.

Gutin, B., Manos, T., Strong, W. (1992). Defining health and fitness: First step toward establishing children's fitness standards. *Research Quarterly for Exercise and Sport, 63* (2), 128–132.

Francis, P. & Francis, L. (1988). *If it hurts don't do it.* Rocklin, CA: Prima Press.

Hoeger, W. W. K., & Hoeger, S. A. (1993). *Fitness and Wellness* (2nd. ed.). Englewood, CO: Morton Publishing.

Haskell, W. L., Leon, A. S., Caspersen, C. J., Victor, F. F., Hagberg, J. M., Harlan, W., Holloszy, J. O., Regensteiner, J. G., Thompson, P. D., Washburn, R. A. & Wilson, P. W. F. (1992). Cardiovascular benefits and assessment of physical activity in adults. *Medicine and Science and Sports and Exercise, 24* (6), Supplement, S201–S220.

Johnson, B. L. & Nelson, J. K. (1986). *The Practical Measurement for Evaluation in Physical Education* (4th ed.). New York: Macmillan Publishing.

Kline, G. M., Porcari, J. P., Hintermeister, R., Freedson, P. S., Ward, A., McCarron, R. F., Ross, J., & Rippe, J. M. (1987). Estimation of VO₂ max from a one-mile track walk, gender, age, and body weight. *Medicine and Science in Sports and Exercise, 19* (3), 253–259.

King, A. C., Blair, S. N., Bild, D. E., Dishman, R. K., Dubbert, P. M., Marcus, B. H., Oldridge, N. B. Paffenbarger, Jr., R. S., Powell, K. E., Yeager, K. K. (1992). Determinants of physical activity and interventions in adults. *Medicine and Science in Sports and Exercise, 24* (6), S221–S233.

Robbins, G., Powers, D., & Burgess, S. (1994). *A wellness way of life.* Madison, WI: WCB Brown & Benchmark.

Williams, B. K. & Knight, S. M. (1993). *Healthy for life: Wellness and the art of living.* Pacific Grove, CA: Brooks/Cole Publishing.

but once I had set out, I was already far on my way

—Colette, 1944

CHAPTER 6
The Warm-Up

The warm-up is designed to prepare the body mentally and physically for a workout. Consisting primarily of rhythmic movement and static stretches, a warm-up should precede any type of moderate or intense activity.

The purpose of this chapter is twofold. The first is to help you understand the importance of a gradual warm-up from a practical, as well as a physiological standpoint. The second is to provide examples of safe pre-activity stretches that, when performed properly, will not put strain on the lower back or joints. Effective stretching will increase the elasticity of muscle fibers and reduce the possibility of injury throughout the aerobic portion of the workout.

WHY WARM UP?

When movement begins the central nervous system transmits signals to the heart and lungs, requesting more oxygen. The respiratory and cardiovascular systems respond immediately by increasing the heart rate. As a result, a greater amount of oxygenated blood becomes available and is transported to the working muscles. During this time the body's core temperature rises, gradually warming and increasing the extensibility of the muscles and tendons and reducing joint stiffness. Warm muscles, tendons and joints adapt more quickly to the exercise load and serve to minimize the possibility of injury.

During exercise, it is important that the initial demand for oxygen does not exceed the capability of the cardiorespiratory system. Several minutes are needed for the system to "catch up" to the demands. Plunging into vigorous activity does not give the cardiorespiratory system time to adapt. You may even experience premature fatigue simply by omitting a gradual warm-up. Your heart and lungs are like the motor of a car. Each must be adequately warmed up to avoid costly breakdowns.

Elements of the Warm-Up

A proper warm-up will last for 7–10 minutes and include rhythmic movement and static stretching. Rhythmic movement consists of low intensity activity (like walking or marching) performed through a full range of motion with the specific purpose of circulating oxygenated blood to warm the muscles. Static stretching prepares the muscles and tendons for safe exercise by increasing your ability to move with less resistance through a full range of motion.

STATIC VS BALLISTIC

There are two basic techniques used to stretch muscles: static stretching and ballistic stretching. The word "stretch" may be a misnomer because only static stretches are capable of increasing the length of a given muscle. Ballistic stretching actually elicits a reflex that inhibits muscle lengthening. **Ballistic stretching** consists of *active bobbing or bouncy movements that activate the muscle's protective stretch reflex mechanism, causing it to contract prematurely and inhibits further gains in the range of motion.* The **stretch reflex** is *designed to protect the muscles, tendons and joints from injury when movements are very rapid and/or uncontrolled.* Ballistic "stretching" serves no real purpose when the goal is to increase the length of a given muscle or muscle group. Further, active bobbing or bouncing places unnecessary stress on the body and is associated with a higher risk of injury. In contrast a **static stretch** is *the slow controlled extension of a muscle to its full length.* Lengthening should continue to the "point of tension" rather than strain. When performing a static stretch work within your own comfort zone. Each stretch should be challenging, yet tolerable. If the position is unbearable, ease back to a more comfortable point. Ideally, this type of stretch is held for 30–60 seconds and is followed by a few seconds of relaxation. Static stretching is not only preferred, it is recommended.

GUIDELINES FOR A SAFE AND EFFECTIVE WARM-UP

1. Begin each warm-up with several minutes of rhythmic movement. Be sure to warm-up the muscles and tendons supporting the knees, by walking or marching, before you perform lateral movements like grapevines or side movements on the step. Remember, cold muscles are less flexible and are more susceptible to tears and strains.

2. Consider the range of motion to be used during the upcoming activity. Stretches performed in conjunction with the warm-up should prepare the body for that activity rather than target overall flexibility. During the warm-up, hold stretches for a minimum of 30 seconds, but avoid overextending. If the muscles begin to "quiver", release the tension a few degrees.

3. Stretch the major muscle groups that are specific to the activity. The following areas of the body may be stretched before an aerobic workout: calves, shins, thighs, torso, upper back, shoulders, and neck.

4. Stretching should never be forced beyond the normal range of motion of the joints. The nor-mal range of motion varies for each individual depending on age, gender and body structure.

5. While stretching, develop an awareness of each muscle group being stretched and relaxed.

6. During static stretching concentrate on breathing (in through the nose before each stretch and out through the mouth) as you hold each position. Holding your breath creates additional tension.

7. Do not allow more than 15 minutes between the completion of the warm-up and the start of your physical activity or the benefits of warming up will be lost.

8. Flexibility may be limited due to a previous physical injury to the joints or muscles. Be sure to work within your limits.

9. Never substitute an analgesic agent such as "Deep Heat" or "Ben-Gay" for a warm-up. These agents create a superficial sensation of warmth that does not penetrate to the deep muscle.

PROPER PRE-ACTIVITY STRETCHING

To prepare the body for more strenuous activity, pre-activity stretches incorporate a minimum range of motion and are often performed while standing. The stretching exercises depicted on the following pages were chosen with care. The debate over "safe" and *contraindicated exercises* is so great that

DON'T

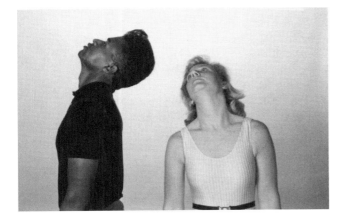

Avoid hyperextending the neck. Avoid head circles as these movements may place unnecessary stress on the cervical vertebrae.

DO

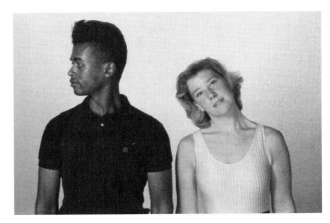

Neck stretches: *targets the **trapezius** and other muscles supporting the head.* Rotate the head gently to each side and hold. Facing the front and keeping both shoulders down, bring the ear toward the shoulder and relax.

DON'T

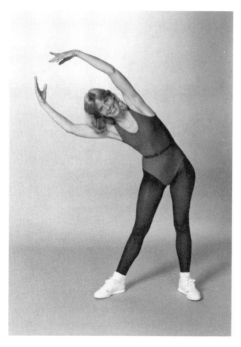

Avoid raising both arms above the head as this places stress on the low back and can force the hip out of alignment. **Avoid** locking the knees. **Avoid** leaning too far to the side.

DO

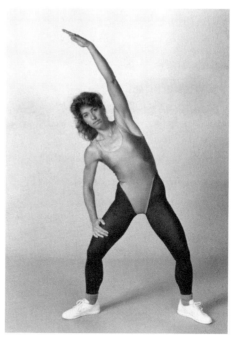

Torso stretch: *targets the* **obliques** *and* **latissimus dorsi**. Stand feet apart, knees slightly bent. Place one hand on the thigh to support the spine. Lift up and extend.

DON'T

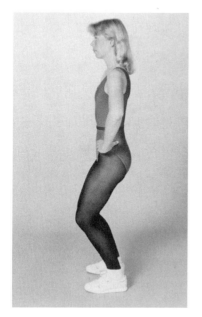

Avoid tilting the pelvis forward. **Avoid** dropping the knees past the toes.

DO

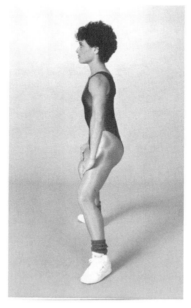

Inner thigh stretches: *targets* **adductors.** Carefully rotate the knees outward while in a squat position.

or

DO

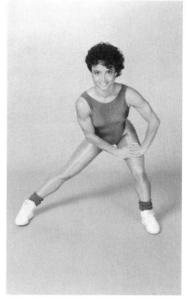

Lunge to the side, keeping both knees slightly bent. Support upper body with hands on thigh.

DON'T   **DO**

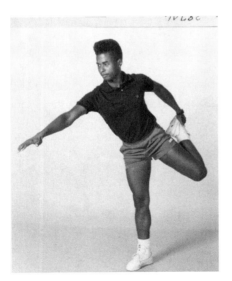

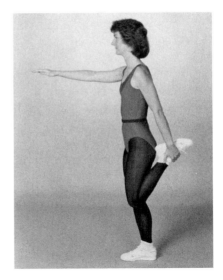

<u>Avoid</u> locking the supporting leg. <u>Avoid</u> arching the back. <u>Avoid</u> grasping the toes with your hands.

Thigh stretch: *targets the* **hip flexors** *and* **quadriceps.** Grasp lower leg and hold near the back of the hip. Keep supporting leg slightly bent. Keep hips square with neck and shoulders relaxed. Careful of the knee joint. *Option: bending the leg but not holding the foot.*

DON'T   **DO**

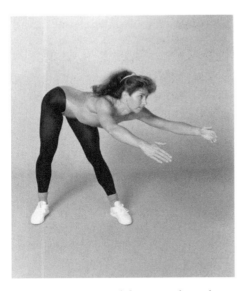

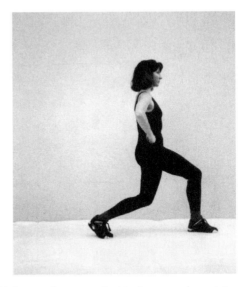

<u>Avoid</u> unsupported forward flexion and standing stretches as these place undo stress on the low back. <u>Avoid</u> hyperextending the neck.

Thigh stretch: *targets the* **hip flexors** *and* **quadriceps.** Start in a forward lunge position. Lift the back heel and tuck the pelvis under. A deeper stretch can be achieved by lowering the body.

DON'T

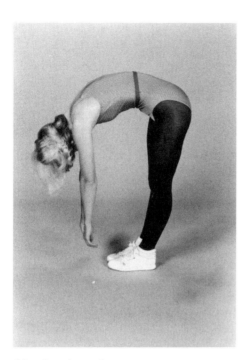

DO

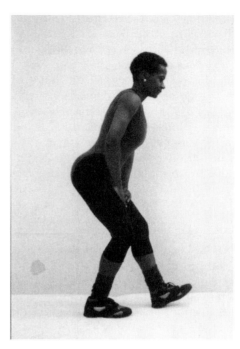

<u>Avoid</u> bending forward; not everyone is strong or flexible enough to maintain that position without strain. <u>Avoid</u> rounding the back. <u>Avoid</u> locking the knees.

Leg stretch: *targets the* **hamstrings** *and* **gluteal muscles.** Keeping your knees close together, flex one foot and extend the leg forward. Lean at the hips and support the upper body with your hands on the thighs.

DO

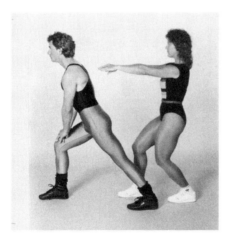

DO

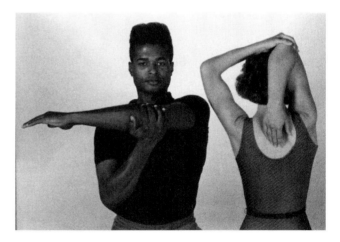

Calf stretch: targets the gastrocnemius. In a forward lunge position, press back heel to the floor. **Calf stretch:** targets the soleus. With one leg slightly forward bend the knees keeping both heels on the floor.

Shoulder stretch: *targets the* **rotator cuff, rhomboids,** *and* **posterior deltoid.** Bring the arm across the body, grasping above the elbow and gently pull toward the body. **Arm stretch:** *targets the* **tricep** *and* **latissimus dorsi.** Raise the arm close to the ear and bend at the elbow. With other hand, gently pull by the elbow and hold. *Option is to use gentle push by the shoulder.*

selections were limited. A **contraindicated exercise** *is an activity that while safe and even effective for a few people is not recommended for the general population.* The splits would be a good example. The hip flexors and hamstrings are stretched during the splits and some people can safely and comfortably manage this position; however, there are several less compromising exercises that are just as effective for stretching those muscles and much safer. Contraindicated exercises pose more risk than benefit, but by substituting alternative activities neither safety nor effectiveness have to be compromised.

In the previous outline we have attempted to show stretches that are commonly used during the warm-up segment of class and "safe" for the general population. Target muscles have been identified so you know where to "feel" the stretch. Common mistakes and contraindicated positions have also been outlined to help you understand technique, proper alignment, and to minimize strain to joints and soft tissue. You may notice that some exercises you once performed are no longer considered the best way to stretch your muscles. In addition, now that you know that ballistic stretching is not effective for flexibility training, you may also have to resist the temptation to bounce, even though "you may have always stretched that way."

The stretches described here are also appropriate to include during the final cool down portion of any workout. In fact, it is recommended that you stretch to increase flexibility after exercising rather than at the beginning. Additional stretches to help promote overall flexibility have been included in chapter 9.

SUMMARY

The warm-up period is essential if exercise is to be safe and effective. A gradual warm-up begins with the rhythmic movement of the large muscles followed by static stretching. Don't stretch before you warm-up! The warm-up prepares the body both physically and mentally for the more strenuous aspects of the workout. Static stretching is the safest and most effective technique to lengthen muscles and tendons to their full range of motion, thus enhancing performance and minimizing joint stiffness and the possibility of injury. Static stretches should also be incorporated during the final portion of each workout.

GLOSSARY

Ballistic Stretching—active bobbing or bouncy movements which inhibit muscle lengthening due to activation of the stretch reflex; not an effective technique for stretching.

Contraindicated Exercise—those activities that may be safe for some but are not recommended for the general population; best avoided by providing participants with a safer, alternative movement.

Rhythmic Movement—consists of low intensity activity (like walking or marching) performed through a full range of motion.

Static Stretching—a slow controlled extension of various muscles or muscle groups to full length, i.e., to the point of tension or stretch tightness. The stretch is ideally held for 30 seconds to one minute and should be followed by a few seconds of relaxation.

Stretch Reflex—one of the body's protective reflex mechanisms which causes a muscle to contract prematurely in an effort to protect itself against injury. This reflex is activated by ballistic movements.

REFERENCES

Anderson, B. (1980). *Stretching.* Bolinas, CA: Shelter Publications, Inc.

Cornelius, W. L. (1990). Flexibility exercise: benefits from flexibility exercise. *National Strength and Conditioning Association Journal, 12* (5), 61–64.

National Strength and Conditioning Association (ed.). (1984). Roundtable: Flexibility. *National Strength and Conditioning Association Journal, Aug.–Sept.*, 10–22, 71–72.

Those who do not find time to exercise will have to find time for illness.

—The Earl of Derby, 1873

CHAPTER 7

Exercise Prescription

The prescription for aerobic exercise is the key to achieving and maintaining good cardiovascular health. The prescription contains three important ingredients: frequency, intensity and duration. These work **in combination** to elicit all of the physiological and psychological benefits discussed in the first chapter of this book. If any one of these ingredients is missing or compromised, the prescription's potency is reduced and the potential benefits are lessened. Total fitness is the result of carefully structuring a program to maximize the benefits. In describing the way the "ingredients" interact, you will understand how to devote your time during exercise.

The purpose of this chapter, therefore, is to present a closer look at the ingredients. It is our hope that a thorough understanding of each will convince you to include all three in your aerobic exercise regime. Then, and only then, will the time and effort you have devoted how to the experience pay off. And the "pay-offs" are well worth it!

FREQUENCY (HOW OFTEN?)

Frequency *refers to the number of days a week you must exercise to achieve the training effect.* The **minimum** is three with the recommended **maximum** six, so that your body receives a day of rest each week. If you opt for the three day a week minimum, be advised that these days should not be consecutive ones. Instead, the three days should be evenly spaced throughout the week, i.e. Monday, Wednesday, Friday or Saturday; or Tuesday, Thursday, Saturday or Sunday. This is due to the unfortunate fact that physical fitness is only temporary. The training effect may start to diminish as quickly as 48 hours after a workout.

When choosing the number of days you plan to exercise each week, it is important to use precaution and common sense. If you are just beginning an aerobic exercise program, start slowly with just two days a week. Increase the frequency very gradually. If you are serious about getting in shape and staying in shape you have the rest of your life to do so. There is no sense trying to undo the effects of years of neglect in a week or a month because it cannot be done safely nor effectively. For general fitness, an every other day schedule seems to offer the best return for the time invested. For weight loss or weight control, however, a five or six day a week schedule is more effective. Yet six days of impact or weight-bearing aerobics, such as jogging or aerobic dance, may lead to overuse injuries for someone just beginning a fitness program. It would be wise, therefore, to choose non weight bearing activities, such as swimming or bicycling, or alternate them with the others. Put into practice the old cliche "everything in moderation."

Beginning aerobic participants, those who have never fully experienced the positive benefits of a regular program, often experience difficulty meeting the frequency requirement. It is so easy to find excuses **not** to exercise. The list of these excuses is endless, but, as stated previously, fitness is not attainable unless prioritized. To achieve success, you must find a way to make exercise a habit, something you do without really thinking about it, so that you don't talk yourself out of it. This will take some experimentation on your part. First, you must try exercising at different times of the day so you can find a time that is best for you.

Morning people find exercise a great way to start their day. It helps them wake up, gives them time to think through the day ahead and seems to get everything started on a positive note. Practically speaking, it means taking a shower and making oneself presentable only once a day and it relieves the pressure of "thinking" about having to exercise during the rest of the day. Too much thinking can get some people into trouble because that is the mechanism used to manufacture the excuses that prevent them from exercising. One excuse leads to another and soon the beginner has abandoned the program without giving it a fair trial.

People who are not early risers or those who cannot realistically fit a morning workout into their schedule have other options. Many choose to work out during their lunch hour, especially if shower facilities are available. Others, who find themselves mentally exhausted or highly stressed at the end of the work day, discover that exercise gives them energy and eventually enhances the quality of their life "after hours". Some people choose to work out later in the evening or before bedtime. Others cannot do so because the rise in metabolism and increase in energy makes it difficult for them to fall asleep.

It is not always easy to find a time to work out that is compatible with your metabolism, schedule and lifestyle. Compromises must often be made. The important thing when beginning an aerobic exercise program is to schedule it a week in advance and stick to that schedule, as if your life depended on it, so that it has a chance of becoming habitual. Many adults join fitness clubs and attend aerobic classes regularly. College students find registering for aerobics classes on campus a good way to begin and maintain an exercise program. Unfortunately, many of these classes only meet 2 or 3 days a week and may not meet your personal need for exercise. If the frequency requirement in the prescription of exercise is going to be met, students should be advised to register for two classes, on alternate days or, better yet, learn to discipline themselves to complete a third or fourth workout on their own. Suggestions and forms for completing self initiated workouts can be found in Appendix B.

Frequency is really the most important ingredient in the prescription. Intensity and duration cannot improve fitness if the exercise is not performed regularly. Even regular exercise will not yield some results for 8–12 weeks.

INTENSITY (HOW HARD?)

Intensity *refers to the amount of effort exerted during exercise or simply, how hard the heart must work to sustain a given workload.* To realize the physical fitness benefits (described in Chapter 1) it is necessary to stress the heart at a prescribed minimum level, which is quantitatively described as 60% of your maximum effort. If, on the other hand, you overload the heart (90–100% effort), you run the risk of overexertion and the exercise shifts from an aerobic to an anaerobic state. **Anaer-**

obic means *"without oxygen"* in the literal sense. Anaerobic exercise is described as high in intensity and short in duration, such as a 100 meter sprint. True anaerobic exercise has a high exhaustion factor and, because it utilizes energy already stored in the muscles (glycogen) it can only be continued for short periods of time. Once the stored energy is used up, the activity can no longer be sustained at a maximum level. In order for the activity to continue, the intensity must be lowered. This enables the cardiorespiratory systems to deliver oxygen (aerobic metabolism) which is needed for the conversion of stored fats to usable energy. The aerobic metabolism allows the exercise to continue for long periods of time and utilizes stored fat in part of the energy process. Many people believe that the harder they work, the more fat they will burn. Such is not the case. Exercising at a moderate rather than exhaustive pace results in fat being utilized as the primary source of energy in the muscles. The "training effect" of exercise is also associated with moderate activity, reinforcing the importance of monitoring physical effort. Three convenient ways to monitor intensity during aerobic activity are training heart rate, a talk test, or perceived exertion.

Calculating Your Training Heart Rate

The most precise way to monitor intensity is to track your pulse for six or ten seconds during exercise or immediately after. This is your training or working heart rate and is measured in beats per minute. A recommended range of intensity has been established for a moderate exercise program, with the **training heart rate zone** *at approximately 60–85% of a person's maximum heart rate.* Your *maximum heart rate* (MHR) is based on your age. By subtracting your current age from 220 you can determine your MHR. The expression "220-age" represents the *maximum number of times your heart will beat in 1 minute.* As your age increases your maximum heart rate decreases such that adjustments in the maximum heart rate will have to be made with each passing year.

Your individual training heart zone can be calculated using your age, resting heart rate, and the appropriate intensity. As you have already monitored and averaged your resting heart rate, you could manually calculate your working heart rate using Karvonen formula:

220 − age − Resting HR × 60–75% + Resting HR = Training heart rate zone.

However, the chart in table 7-1 has already computed individual training zone based on resting

TABLE 7-1

Training Heart Rate Zone

(based on the Karvonen formula and 60–80% of maximum heart rate)

Average Resting Heart		Less than 25	25–29	30–34	35–39	40–44	45–49	50–54	55–59	60–64	Over 65
below 50	Target zone	136–166	133–164	130–160	127–156	124–152	121–148	118–144	115–140	112–136	109–134
50–54	Target zone	138–167	135–165	132–161	129–157	126–153	123–149	120–145	117–141	114–137	111–135
55–59	Target zone	140–168	137–166	134–162	131–158	128–154	125–150	122–146	119–142	116–138	113–136
60–64	Target zone	142–169	139–167	136–163	133–159	130–155	127–151	124–147	121–143	118–139	115–137
65–69	Target zone	144–170	141–168	138–164	135–160	132–156	129–152	126–148	123–144	120–140	117–138
70–74	Target zone	146–171	143–169	140–165	137–161	134–157	131–153	128–149	125–145	122–141	119–139
75–79	Target zone	148–172	145–170	142–166	139–162	136–158	133–154	130–150	127–146	124–142	121–140
80–85	Target zone	150–173	147–171	144–167	141–163	138–159	135–155	132–151	129–147	126–143	123–141
86 and over	Target zone	152–174	149–172	146–168	143–164	140–160	137–156	134–152	131–148	128–144	125–142

Adapted from Corbin, C. B., & Lindsey, R. (1994). *Concepts of physical fitness with laboratories.* (8th ed.) Dubuque, IA: Wm C. Brown.

heart rate and age. During class occasional pulse checks can be taken to help you monitor intensity. You find your working pulse rate in the same manner used to locate your resting heart (as described in chapter 1). If after taking your pulse rate you find that it is below your training zone, you can safely increase your pace. In contrast, if your heart rate is above your recommended training zone, you should modify your intensity. Chapter 8 will provide you with guidelines for intensity modification.

The chart in table 7-1 is different from what you might encounter in health clubs which are based only on age. It is important for students to understand how the formula is designed to accommodate persons with different levels of conditioning. For example, two 20-year-old students will have the same maximum heart rate. But one student may have a resting heart rate of 78 beats per minute, while the other student has a resting heart rate of 60 beats per minute. As you can see, the formula will become individualized as a result of subtracting two different resting heart rates. While the difference may not be very large, it does have an impact on intensity. Using your average resting heart and age, check the chart for your training zone.

The final step is to determine what your training heart rate zone would be for 6 and 10 seconds. For a 6 second count, simply divide your two numbers by 10. Likewise, for a 10 second count, divide both numbers by 6.

Remember, your training heart rate is a function of age, resting heart rate and activity level. It is a good practice to reassess your resting heart rate periodically and adjust for age and activity level as needed. This way, you are sure to be exercising in a range specifically designed for you.

Once you have determined your target heart zone, you can monitor your **working heart rate** (*pulse during exercise*) to see if you are working aerobically. The easiest way to monitor your pulse during exercise is to wear a digital watch that displays the seconds or a watch that has a sweep second hand. You can find your pulse easily using either the radial or carotid artery as described in Chapter 3. Exercise caution when taking the pulse at the carotid artery since excessive pressure can trigger a reflex that slows the heart momentarily. In addition, avoid using the thumb because it has a pulse of its own that could interfere with getting an accurate count. Count your pulse for six seconds and multiply by 10 (add a zero) or count for ten seconds and multiply by 6 to determine the number of beats per minute. Most professionals agree that a 10 second count is more accurate, but a 6 second count is easier to calculate in one's head. In your creative aerobic fitness class, the method you use will be determined by your instructor. Either way, you are advised to begin your counting with 0 since the signal "GO" does not always correspond with the first heart beat you feel. Again, if you discover that the rate per minute is not as high as the lowest end of your training heart zone, you will know to increase the intensity. On the other hand, if your heart rate is too high, you will know to slow down or lessen the intensity. You need not be alarmed if you are over the upper end of your heart zone if you feel fine both during and after exercise. You should be concerned only if there are signs of over-exertion, such as:

- Extreme difficulty breathing
- A heart rate in excess of 120 beats per minute that persists 5 to 10 minutes after the activity has stopped
- Fatigue that lasts up to 24 hours after the activity has stopped
- Extreme muscle soreness or muscle cramps that persist for days
- Difficulty sleeping at night

Talk Test

In addition to monitoring your working heart rate you can use the **talk-test** to gage your general intensity. A *moderately paced workout will allow you to breathe and still carry on a conversation with a friend*. This indicates that adequate oxygen is being delivered to the working muscles. Of course, if you can sing the *Star Spangled Banner*, you are probably not working hard enough. When you first increase your intensity you may feel a little tired, but you should not feel breathless for very long. If at any-time during class you do feel breathless, use this feedback and decrease your intensity to a more moderate pace.

Rating Perceived Exertion

Another convenient way to monitor your inten-sity is by estimating how you feel. This is called **Rate of Perceived Exertion** and it *is a subjective measure of intensity that with practice can be a very effective means of gaging your effort*. It is not always convenient to take a heart rate and in most cases heart rates are taken infrequently during class. By asking yourself "how you feel" you can gauge your intensity anytime during your workout. The Borg scale was the first attempt at developing a subjec-tive but reliable means for measuring exercise effort. This 6–20 point scale was designed to corre-spond with the actual training heart of exercise subjects; however, the subjects were in their twen-ties and the scale is skewed to younger participants. Table 7-2 is a modified version of this scale. Partici-pants should attempt to work between 6–8 to achieve a moderate intensity. An intensity of 9 or 10 represents an exhaustive effort and is neither necessary nor recommended for general fitness development.

TABLE 7-2

Perceived Exertion

On a scale of 1 to 10, how do **you** feel when you're working out?

10 — Maximal Effort
9 — Peaking
8 — CHALLENGING
7 — TRAINING
6 — CONDITIONING
5 — Warming-up/Cooling down
4 — Moving
3 — Standing
2 — Resting
1 — Sleeping

How to Use Perceived Exertion to Monitor Your Intensity

Think of these numbers as the effort you are using to maintain your current activity. Consider how hard you are breathing, muscu-lar fatigue, body temperature, and any other sensations you notice resulting from your exercise. Understand that general fitness and cardiovascular conditioning are not based on giving 100%. All you need to do is challenge yourself at a comfortable pace. With practice perceived exertion can be a very reliable indi-cator of intensity. It is also more convenient than taking a pulse rate and can be taken anytime without interrupting your workout.

So how hard you are you working out? YOU BE THE JUDGE!

Designed by Jennifer Park and adapted from Borg, G. A. V. (1982). Psychophysical bases of per-ceived exertion. *Medicine and Science in Sports and Exercise, 14,* 380.

Your **recovery heart rate,** which should be taken several times after you stop exercising, *is another way to measure the intensity of your workout and is also an indication of your fitness level*. People who are physically fit generally recover more quickly than those who are not because their cardiorespira-tory systems are more efficient and able to adapt more easily to the extra workload. A recovery heart rate taken one minute after exercise should yield a rapid decrease from the working rate. Five minutes after exercise, the heart rate should be 120 beats per minute or less. Ten minutes afterward it should be below 100 beats per minute. Thirty minutes afterward it should be close to the pre exercise rate. When this occurs, you know you are exercising safely. You should find yourself sleeping well at night and waking refreshed. Any tightness or muscle soreness you experience should diminish during your next exercise session.

DURATION (HOW LONG?)

Duration *refers to the length of time you must engage in non stop aerobic exercise.* There are two basic approaches to gaging duration of aerobic exercise. One is to participate in a single continuous bout of activity for approximately twenty to sixty minutes. The other method is **intermittent exercise** and *involves a short duration of activity repeated several times during the day.* The duration of activity depends on several factors, including the goal of the program, the intensity of the activity, and the time available to exercise. If the goal of the program is weight loss, the intensity of the activity should be low to moderate and time not limited. A single continuous bout of exercise 20–60 minutes in length would be recommended. However, if cardiovascular conditioning is the primary goal, a moderate to high intensity activity can be planned, or if time is simply limited, then an intermittent program can provide the benefits desired.

To maximize fat burning and weight control, most experts recommend at least 20 minutes of continuous exercise that is vigorous enough to get the heart rate within the training zone and keep it there. Moderate activities sustained for 30–60 minutes are even more suited for weight loss. For maintaining cardiovascular conditioning when time is limited an intermittent approach to exercise will contribute to your fitness. Ten minute exercise sessions repeated two or more times a day will contribute comparable cardiovascular benefits as exercising continuously for a longer duration. Your goal is to *accumulate* 20 minutes of activity in a day. Busy individuals having difficulty finding an hour every day for an exercise class can use this exercise prescription. When time is limited take a few minutes to climb an extra flight of stairs or walk a little farther on your way to class. Consider that if you do ten minutes of exercise in the morning, then again during lunch and later in the evening, you will have accumulated 30 minutes of activity by the end of the day. This is not the ideal exercise prescription for weight loss, but will help keep you fit.

MODE

Mode *refers to the type of activity that is generally considered to be aerobic.* For a complete list, refer to Chapter 1. In general, to be labeled "aerobic" the activity must be performed continuously and use the legs. Stopping and starting activities such as tennis or racquetball do **not** strictly qualify when played according to the rules. To be aerobic, a rally must be sustained for as long as possible and, when interrupted, the players must keep their feet moving by jogging in place, or running to retrieve balls that are no longer in play.

Aerobic exercises must also be vigorous enough to get the heart rate into the individually prescribed training zone and keep it there for the 20 minute duration. Thus, acceptable activities will vary among individuals. Less fit individuals may satisfy the intensity requirement with brisk walking or non-impact aerobics. More fit individuals may need to choose jogging, running, low-impact or high-impact aerobics instead.

Creative aerobic fitness programs are designed for people of all ages and fitness levels because the responsibility for the intensity of the workout ultimately rests with the student. Qualified instructors help by providing numerous examples of ways to modify steps at low, medium and high levels of intensity. But it is up to each participant to monitor their pulse at regular spaced intervals to insure that they are exercising within their individually prescribed training heart zones.

PRESCRIPTION FOR EXERCISE

INTENSITY (HOW HARD?)	=	60–85% of your maximum heart rate
DURATION (HOW LONG?)	=	20–60 minutes continuous or 20 minutes accumulated through intermittent exercise
FREQUENCY (HOW OFTEN?)	=	3 times per week (minimum)

OVERLOAD PRINCIPLE

When you first begin an aerobic program you will find that your heart rate and your breathing increase sharply. But with repetition and regular participation over a period of time your body will adapt to the increased workload. As your heart, lungs and muscles begin to function more efficiently your fitness level will improve. You are able to complete a given workout with less exertion. This is known as the **overload principle.** Simply stated, your *body adapts to greater workloads than it is accustomed to and eventually increases its capacity to do more work.* Thus, continual improvement of the cardiovascular system will require increased demands on the heart and lungs. This can be achieved by increasing the frequency, intensity and/or duration. You may find that you have to work harder (walk more briskly, run faster, etc.) to raise your heart rate to its training zone. That is why it is important to monitor your heart rate periodically, even after the 8–12 week break-in period.

You may also feel like working out more often (increasing the frequency) or prolonging the length of each workout session (increasing the duration) as your program progresses. With each change, your body adapts and you acquire a greater level of fitness. But remember, the reverse is also true. If you reduce your level of activity or cut back on your program you reduce your fitness level. This, in fact, can occur rather quickly. A good rule of thumb is to let your body be your guide. When it feels right to do more, do it. Just don't over do it or overload too quickly. You want to achieve the training effect with little or no discomfort.

SUMMARY

The prescription for aerobic exercise, when followed in its entirety, has the potential to change your life. It necessitates performing an activity **at least** 3 times a week (frequency) that raises your heart rate to your individually prescribed training zone (intensity) and accumulating at least 20 minutes (duration) of activity either continuously or intermittently. Developing and maintaining a safe and effective aerobic fitness program requires time, effort and most of all, commitment. You **can** do it. It may help if you change "have to" into "want to". When you decide you want all or some of the benefits described in Chapter 1, write yourself a prescription and get started. It is never too late to discover the joys of fitness and experience them for the remainder of your life.

GLOSSARY

Aerobic—"with oxygen"—the aerobic system depends upon the delivery and utilization of oxygen for prolonged activity.

Anaerobic—"without oxygen"—the anaerobic system is a short term, limited system that provides an immediate source of energy for bursts of intense activity.

Duration—refers to the length of time a person is engaged in continuous aerobic exercise (20 minutes or more is recommended).

Frequency—refers to the number of days a week you must exercise to achieve the training effect. The minimum is 3 and the recommended maximum is 6.

Intensity—the amount of effort expended during exercise. It is expressed as a percentage of your maximum heart rate.

Intermittent Exercise—a short bout (5–10 minutes) of activity followed by rest and another short bout of exercise; several independent sessions of activity performed for a short period of time.

Maximum Heart Rate—(220—Age) The maximum number of times the heart will beat in one minute.

Mode—type of activity.

Overload Principle—placing more stress on a muscle than it normally encounters in daily use in an effort to improve the components of health related physical fitness.

Rate of Perceived Exertion—a way to monitor your intensity is by estimating how you feel; a subjective measure of intensity that with practice can be a very effective means of gaging your effort.

Recovery Heart Rate—heart rate taken at least five minutes after exercise has ceased. Cooldown is complete when recovery heart is 120 bpm or less.

Talk-Test—a method for monitoring general intensity; a moderately paced workout will allow you to breathe and still carry on a conversation with a friend.

Training Heart Rate Zone—a safe and effective heart rate zone for exercising aerobically that is 60–85% of a person's maximum heart rate.

Working Heart Rate—heart rate taken during or immediately following aerobic exercise.

REFERENCES

American College of Sports Medicine. (1991). *Guidelines for exercise testing and prescription* (4th ed.). Philadelphia: Lea & Febiger.

Dunbar, C. C., Robertson, R. J., Baun, R., Blandin, M. F., Metz, K., Burdett, R., & Goss, F. L. (1992). The validity of regulating exercise intensity by ratings of perceived exertion. *Medicine and Science in Sports and Exercise, 24* (1), 94–99.

Entzion, K. L. & Whitehead, J. R. (1993). A comparison of two methods of teaching appropriate intensity of cardiovascular exercise: Manually measured heart rates and perception of perceived exertion. *Research Quarterly in Exercise and Sport.*

Nelson, D. J., Pels, A. E., Geenen, D. L., & White, T. P. (1988). Cardiac frequency and caloric cost of aerobic dancing in young women. *Research Quaterly for Exercise and Sport, 59* (3), 229–233.

There is a vitality, a life force, an energy, a quickening that is translated through you into action . . . dance your story.

–Martha Graham

CHAPTER 8

Aerobics in Action

Cardiovascular activity is the core of the creative aerobic fitness program. This phase of the program consists primarily of basic locomotor skills (walk, run, jump, hop, skip, and slide), combinations of these skills (step-hop, walk-jump, etc.), and other movements derived from dance (chause, grapevine, mamba, cha cha cha, etc.). All of these skills are dynamic movements using large muscles that are performed to music with the purpose of elevating the heart rate and promoting cardiovascular endurance.

Aerobic dance has gone through many changes since it was first introduced by Jackie Sorenson in 1969. It is likely that more changes will follow. Aerobic dance was first labelled a fitness trend: a popular activity but not likely to last. After more than two decades aerobic dance is still a popular activity. The evolution has included high impact classes, then low impact, and followed by classes that integrate both. Teaching styles have also changed. Structured choreography was followed by spontaneous freestyle movements and then pattern recall and progressive routines. Changes have also followed popular music styles. Hip hop, country, Latin sounds and even disco have inspired instructors and participants to move in new and different ways.

The variety of aerobic dance, both past and present, is evident of the flexible nature of this exercise medium. The enduring and evolving nature of aerobic dance is a result of the changing needs and interest of the participants. Knowledge of the many different styles of aerobics, as well as, how to modify intensity and movements will help you find the activity that best suits you.

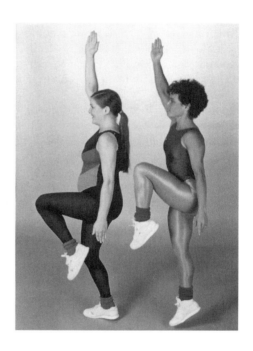

AEROBIC TECHNIQUE

Cardiovascular conditioning is the product of continuous movement, specifically continuous movement of the lower body. As discussed in chapter 1 many different modes of exercise can be employed to promote cardiovascular fitness, including swimming, cycling, and cross country skiing. Movement variety is also a component of aerobic dance. There are two distinct movement techniques used in aerobic dance and several variations thereof. High-impact and low-impact are the foundation of a creative aerobic fitness program. Integrating techniques, movements and intensity modifications are additional topics to be outlined in this chapter. Aerobic programs incorporating step activities and slide training will be discussed in Chapter 10.

Traditional Aerobics

Traditional or high-impact aerobics *utilizes a variety of locomotor and dance skills with an identifiable* *flight phase during the movements.* With each hop and jump the body's **center of gravity** is elevated and lowered, generating the momentum that challenges skeletal muscles and conditions the heart. Generally, both feet leave the floor at the same time. There is often repetition of quick ballistic movements that creates a spring-back or rebound effect upon impact with the floor. It is important not to dance on the toes but to land using the entire foot, rolling down from the ball of the foot through the heel. Those who choose proper footwear and/or those who use proper landing techniques seldom incur injuries to the lower extremities. Such injuries are usually a result of poor alignment, improper footwear, incorrect technique or overuse. We recommend utilization of all three impact variations within a given class so that you may adapt the workout to meet your individual needs.

While many people can enjoy performing high impact movements, recommendations have been made concerning movement repetition. Jumping jacks should be limited to eight repetitions and should be followed by movements that change impact forces. Movements incorporating single foot landings, such as repetitive knee lifts on the right leg, should also be limited to eight or less repetitions before changing legs or movements. Safety and effectiveness also depends on *movement follow through.* **Movement follow-through** *in aerobic dance is essential, minimizing the landing forces and preparing the body for the next skill.* This consists of bending the knees and rolling through the foot with each landing. Without follow-through the momentum of each movement is lost and flow stilted, the result is movements that are jerky.

Low-Impact Aerobics

Low-impact aerobics *centers around movements that keeps one foot on the floor most of the time, thus limiting the overall landing forces.* Like high-impact, low-impact movements also involve raising and lowering of the center of gravity, but rather than jumping, more flexion and extension is produced by the knees. Also, each step is accompanied by a controlled landing rather than a rebound. Low-impact movements usually incorporate more traveling and directional changes than traditional high impact aerobics. So in addition to raising and lowering the center of gravity, the body is also propelled horizontally. Intensity is derived not from the vertical jumps or hops, but rather bending and extending the knees and horizontal traveling. Combining these two techniques can provide a

very challenging workout while minimizing impact to the body.

Most participants use low-impact as a means for achieving a challenging cardiovascular workout while minimizing the stress to the lower body. However, there are safety concerns even for low-impact participants. If repetitive knee flexion and extension aggravates the knee, these movements should be minimized. However, intensity can still be sustained by using traveling and directional changes. Also, working out on carpeted surfaces increases the friction between the floor and the foot. While traveling during low impact, conscious effort must be taken not to shuffle feet which may cause soreness in knees and ankles. Instead the foot up must be purposefully lifted with each step.

A qualified instructor will model different variations within a workout, but it is up to the participants to monitor their heart rate and modify their movements so that they can continue to exercise within their training heart zones.

Integrated Aerobics

Classes utilizing both high and low impact movements are one of the most common aerobic classes available. **Integrated aerobics** *are movement patterns that utilize both high and low impact aerobics.* These classes are an effective way to accommodate the different interests and needs of a variety of participants. Any aerobic class offered at a health club, recreational facility, or even college will attract students of different fitness levels and experience. Even labeling a class beginning, intermediate, or advanced won't preclude anyone joining. Many people involve themselves in activities that are convenient rather than appropriate for their needs. That is, if a class is offered at a convenient time and place, a variety of people will show up. Integrated aerobics coupled with knowledge of intensity modification will allow people with different skills, fitness levels and physical needs to successfully engage in the same aerobics class.

Integrated classes may be presented in two distinct ways. The first is to demonstrate high-impact movements while showing low-impact modifications. Another is to use a single routine that incorporates some high-impact and some low-impact movements together, showing additional movement modifications for those who may require them.

Regardless of the impact level or combinations chosen for a workout, it is important to begin the aerobic portion at a low intensity by utilizing small movements of the major muscle groups. As the workout continues, the intensity level should increase until you are working within your training heart rate zone. Remember, during an aerobic dance class, once the target heart rate is reached, you want to keep it there for at least 20 minutes to achieve the maximum benefits. The intensity should decrease gradually as you approach the cool down phase of the workout.

POSTURAL AND ALIGNMENT CONSIDERATIONS

While exercising aerobically, it is important to practice the principles of good posture and breathing discussed in Chapter 4. Reminders and cautions are listed below.

DON'T

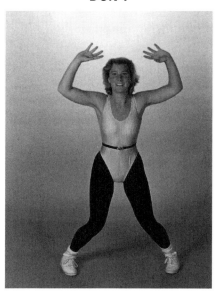

<u>Avoid</u> rotating the knees and toes inward.

DO

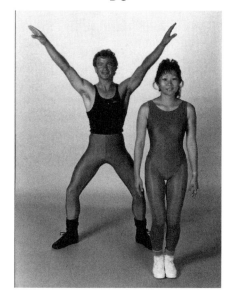

Keep knees above and in line with the direction of the toes. Bend the knees with each landing.

DON'T

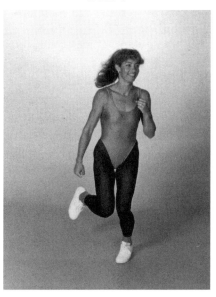

<u>Avoid</u> rotating the feet outward when jogging. Heels should lift directly behind leg.

DO

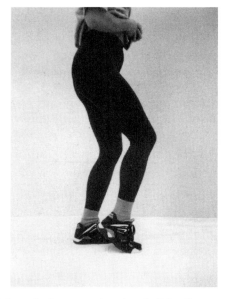

Roll through the entire foot (toe-ball-heel), as each contacts the floor. Make sure your heels contact the floor with every movement.

DON'T

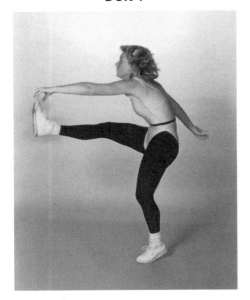

DO

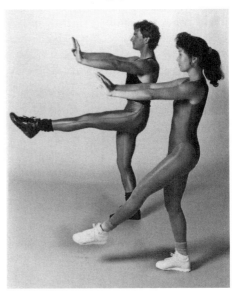

Avoid rounding shoulders and upper back. Avoid tilting pelvis forward or backward. Avoid throwing or flinging your extremities in an uncontrolled manner. Avoid locking your knees.

Keep the back straight with shoulders relaxed. Kick only as high as your flexibility allows. Control your movements. Keep the knees slightly bent at all times.

MOVEMENT MODIFICATIONS VS. INTENSITY MODIFICATIONS

High-impact, low-impact and integrated movements are techniques for moving that can be performed at a variety of intensities. When first introduced, low-impact was an alternative to high impact aerobics and a way to minimize the stress to the body. Unfortunately, low-impact was often considered a less challenging workout. The different impact levels are ways to modify movements but not necessarily intensify. Intensity doesn't have to be sacrificed just because you need to modify impact.

Intensity in high-impact, low-impact and integrated aerobics is related to physical effort and not inherent to a specific technique. In aerobic dance effort is achieved and sustained by:

- raising and lowering of the center of gravity
- moving the center of gravity horizontally
- maintaining strong body position
- using full range of motion
- completing each movement with follow-through.

Music speed and arm movements can also contribute to exercise intensity but with limitations.

Music tempo varies depending on the style of aerobics being performed. Low-impact may use music as slow as 135 beats per minute (bpm), while high-impact can use music as fast as 160 bpm. Faster music used does not necessarily elicit a more effective workout. Trying to keep up with fast music may mean sacrificing technique and using smaller range of motion, especially for tall participants. In contrast many movements are generated by using momentum and may not be well sustained with music at 135 bpm. Music used in the middle ranges is usually most successful for a variety of movements, while still allowing for complete range of motion, movement follow through, and most important control.

Arm movements can contribute to cardiovascular conditioning, but not to the extent that continuous leg movements can. Heart rate does increase with arm movements. However, when the arms are above shoulders the heart has to work harder to pump circulating blood up hill. The result is an increased heart rate and greater perceived exertion. However, research shows that only limited increases in cardiovascular function are achieved with vigorous arm movements. So while intensity can be gained from incorporating upper body movements, the arms should not be emphasized over leg movements.

The most confusing aspect of movement and intensity modifications is that though distinct, they do share common characteristics. Participants needing to modify low impact movements to protect their knees should limit range of motions, while participants who want to decrease intensity may opt to do the same thing. Table 8-1 provides you the specifics of modification.

TEACHING STYLES AND PATTERN DEVELOPMENT

Movement presentation in aerobics depends largely on the preferences and experience of the instructor and the goals of the class. Movement selection and sequencing can vary from the very simple to the complex and from the random to the predetermined.

Aerobics as introduced by Judy Sheppard-Mizzet incorporated **choreographed routines;** *specific movements set to specific music.* Jazzercise™ still uses this method of instruction as its program. Choreographed routines work well with established groups who over time have the opportunity to learn the pattern. New participants may have trouble following at first, but with time will feel very successful.

In contrast to established routines, **freestyle instruction** *incorporates random selection of movements that progressively changes but does not develop into a repeatable pattern.* Freestyle instruction can involve high repetition of movements where the leg pattern remains the same but arms or directions change. Freestyle can be very effective for participants new to aerobics and need to practice movements and transitions.

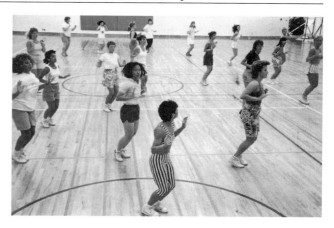

Pattern recall *is a style of teaching where individual movements are presented, practiced, and then combined into progressive routines.* The movements are usually organized into eight-count segments. The two segments or 16 counts are then combined to form a larger teaching module and practiced together. Two new eight count segments are individually introduced and then combined. Finally, both 16 count segments are linked into a 32 count pattern. A longer routine can be developed, using additional 32 count modules. Unlike choreographed routines, pattern recall can be used with most music, and as each routine is developed during class, is less dependent on participant memorizing that develop into routine. With good cuing pattern recall is very effective for all levels of participants.

TABLE 8-1			
Modification for Aerobic Dance			
Technique Characteristics		Intensity	Movements
High Impact uses vertical rebounding with an identifiable flight phase	To decrease	—minimize arm movements —perform less rebounding	—perform less rebounding —decrease range of motion —change impact levels if necessary
	To increase	—increase rebounding —incorporate more travelling	
Low Impact uses controlled movements with minimal flight, incorporating horizontal traveling & knee bends	To decrease	—minimize arm movements —make horizontal movements smaller	—make smaller horizontal movements —raise center of gravity (decrease knee bend) —eliminate any rebounds
	To increase	—lower center of gravity —increase horizontal traveling —add controlled rebounds	

Circuits, Stations and Creative Activities

The goal of a good creative aerobic fitness program is to provide the student with a variety of impact variations and aerobic styles, interspersed with fun and creative ways of achieving cardiovascular fitness. To achieve the latter, circuits, stations and creative activities can be devised that are limited only by the imagination of your instructor.

Circuits are generally circular in nature. Participants establish their own pace as they jog or run from one point to another, stopping only long enough to complete a designated task. An example would be a par course, found in many community parks or recreation areas. The individual tasks are usually pictured and/or described on a sign. Most are designed to enhance the strength or muscular endurance of various muscle groups, although cardiorespiratory endurance remains the overall priority. In creative aerobic fitness classes, tasks can involve strength, muscular endurance and/or aerobic exercises, with the added usage of elastic bands or light weights.

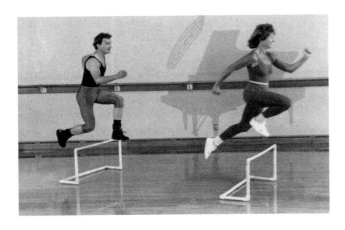

Stations involve a group of students participating in a given task for a specified period of time. Examples of tasks include jogging, leaping over hurdles, jumping rope, following the leader in freestyle aerobics, completing a mini-circuit of exercises, and/or practicing manipulative skills such as dribbling a basketball or soccer ball while on the move. When the time is up, a signal sounds and the entire group rotates to the next station.

Creative activities generally promote interaction among students in a fun and game-like situation. These are activities that do not center around teacher demonstration, but allow students the opportunity to develop their own movements or routines. This can be done in partners, with small groups, and with the entire class following. Such exercises are designed to provide a workout that is spontaneous, interesting and enjoyable, while providing social interaction for participants.

SUMMARY

Aerobic dance offers a versatile approach to cardiovascular fitness, accommodating the interests and fitness levels of a spectrum of participants. High impact, low impact and integrated aerobics are techniques of executing movements, while choreographed, freestyle and pattern recall are styles of teaching and combining movements. Effort and intensity are maintained, regardless of technique or style, by strong/controlled body position, using continuous and full range of motion, movement follow through, and traveling. Music speed and arm movements do contribute to exercise intensity but with limitations and should not be emphasized over control and continuous leg movements. A gradual increase in intensity following warm-up is crucial to a safe and effective workout and is the responsibility.

GLOSSARY

Center of Gravity—the center most point in the body around which all weight is balanced.

Choreography—creating and arranging movement patterns into a specified sequence, usually to a designated piece of music.

Circuit—a circular course with specified tasks to complete en route.

Freestyle Aerobics—a teaching style that is improvisational in nature and uses a combination of movements that logically and progressively build upon each other.

Integrated Aerobics—movement patterns that utilize both high and low impact aerobics; this style of moving is an effective way to accommodate the different interests and needs of a variety of participants.

Intensity Modifications—changes in movements or range of motion that affects the effort of the activity.

Low-Impact Aerobics—centers around movements that keeps one foot on the floor most of the time, thus limiting the overall landing forces.

Movement Follow-Through—in aerobic dance is essential for minimizing the landing forces and preparing the body to produce the next movement; bending the knees and rolling through the foot with each landing.

Movement Modifications—changing or substituting movements so as to prevent discomfort or to increase the level of the skill.

Pattern Recall—is a style of teaching where individual movements are presented, practiced, and then combined into a progressive routine.

Stations—exercise centers that provide an opportunity for small groups of students to work on a designated task for a specified period of time.

Traditional or High-Impact Aerobics—utilizes a variety of locomotor and dance skills with an identifiable flight phase during movement.

REFERENCES

Thomsen, D. & Ballor, D. L. (1991). Physiological Responses during aerobic dance of individuals grouped by aerobic capacity and dance experience. *Research Quarterly for Exercise and Sport,* 62 (1), 68–72.

> *The great end of life is not knowledge but action.*
> —Thomas Henry Huxley, 1825–95

CHAPTER 9
Aerobic Cool Down, Isolated Conditioning, and Final Stretch

In addition to gradual warm-up and cardiovascular conditioning, a complete aerobic class includes an aerobic cool down, isolated conditioning, and a final stretch. Each of these components serve to provide a complete and safe workout. The purpose, basic principles, and safety guidelines of each of these components will be described in this chapter.

AEROBIC COOL DOWN

The **cool down** is designed to decrease the exercise intensity gradually and is defined *as that period of time which immediately follows the aerobic conditioning segment.* During the aerobic workout, blood is circulating rapidly throughout your body. A sudden halt in vigorous exercise will cause the blood to pool at your feet, reducing the flow of blood and oxygen to other parts of the body, particularly your brain. Dizziness and/or fainting may follow.

Cool down activities should include rhythmical movement for the lower body, be designed to decrease heart rate gradually, and be sustained for a minimum of 5 minutes. To ensure that the body sufficiently recovers from activity a recovery heart rate can be taken after the aerobic cool down. A **recovery heart rate** *can be used to monitor cardiovascular intensity (function) after exercise and provides feedback concerning how to proceed with your workout.* When your recovery heart rate reaches 120 beats or less, you can safely stretch and resume other activities or proceed with isolated conditioning such as push ups.

Walking activities should be continued until the recovery heart is achieved. Those just starting a regular aerobic program will take longer to recover from exercise than someone already in condition.

As aerobic fitness improves, less recovery time will be needed. Remember, a rapid recovery from vigorous aerobic exercise is one of the benefits of an aerobic conditioning program.

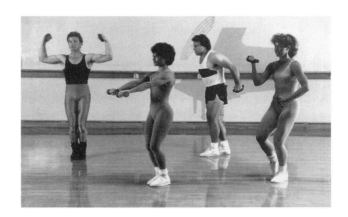

ISOLATED CONDITIONING

Isolated conditioning *includes exercises designed to target specific muscles and muscle groups with the purpose of improving muscular strength and endurance.* Many programs will include isolated conditioning prior to aerobic activity, while other classes may do standing leg work before and additional floor work after aerobics. There are advantages to either format and both are safe and physiologically sound training options as long as they are preceded by a warm-up and followed by stretching.

Specific exercises may vary among instructors, but will generally include those that strengthen the shoulders, arms, upper back, abdomen, hips and legs. Using isometric and isotonic contractions, a variety of exercises can be performed either standing, sitting or lying down. Incorporating equipment such as weights, dynabands, and tubing can increase the resistance and challenge more advanced participants.

An **isometric contraction** *occurs when a muscle contracts but no movement is observed.* In other words, the muscle develops tension but there is no change in the relative length of the limb segments. An example of an isometric contraction would be to stand in a door way, placing both hands against the door jam and pushing as hard as you can. The muscles in your arms produce a significant amount of tension, but no movement results. In contrast, an **isotonic contraction** *is a "dynamic" muscular contraction that produces movement in the corresponding limbs.* All dynamic movements performed by our muscles (lunges, squats and crunches) are considered to be isotonic muscle contractions. Each muscle and/or muscle group can be exercised to its fullest capacity by incorporating both types of muscle contractions. This is achieved by first tightening a muscle or muscle group and then moving the limb through its range of motion. This is the key to body shaping.

Tight and controlled movements with a double emphasis on proper alignment and technique are necessary to achieve strength, endurance and toning benefits. There are several ways to perform many of the isolated exercises. Knowledge of proper alignment, technique, and alternative movements will enable you to perform each exercise safely and effectively. Exercises can be made more challenging by increasing the range of motion, adding resistance, and using more advanced positions. Poor alignment and improper technique render the exercise ineffective, not to mention hazardous. Preventing injury, particularly to the neck and low back,

is a primary concern of the instructor and should be your concern as well. Concentrate on your body position as you exercise and emphasize strong, controlled movements. Do only what you are capable of. If the exercise creates a painful burning sensation and/or cramping develops within the muscle, take a short break to breathe and stretch, then continue with the exercise using correct form. Breathing must be a conscious effort. Breathing is taken for granted by most participants. Unless your instructor reminds you not to hold your breath when the exercise becomes difficult, you probably won't think about it.

ADDING RESISTANCE

Resistance exercises can be easily and safely incorporated into the isolated conditioning segment of class. However, special consideration must be taken before weights are used in conjunction with aerobic activities.

Students may choose to perform strength and muscular endurance exercises with the resistance of their own body weight against the force of gravity, or with additional weight in the form of hand-held or wrist weights, ankle weights or elastic bands. Weight resistance exercises may be performed in conjunction with aerobics or floor-work. Beginners, however, should avoid the use of added weight resistance until the exercise can be accomplished easily without weights. Ankle weights should never be used to perform the aerobic portion of the workout and are directly associated with a high rate of injury to the lower extremity. Caution is also advised when using wrist weights during

DON'T

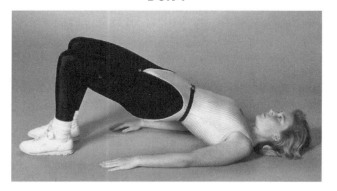

Avoid lifting the back off the ground as this puts pressure on the neck and shoulders. Avoid dropping the chest forward. Avoid lifting up the front heel. Avoid going too low.

DO

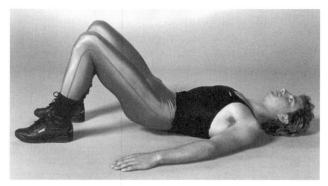

Pelvic tilts: *targets* **abdominals and gluteals.** With knees bent and feet apart contract the muscles in the hips and then relax.

DON'T

DO

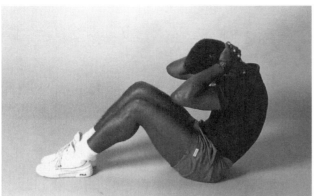

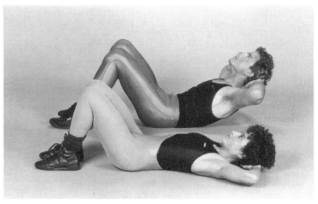

Avoid full sit ups. The exercise primarily works the hips flexors and places unnecessary stress on the low back and neck.

Ab Curl or Crunch: *targets the* **Rectus Abdominus** *and* **Transverse Obliques.** Begin lifting with center of your chest, using your abdominals. Keep your back pressed to the floor, your elbows relaxed, and your head relaxed in hands. Exhale as you lift up.

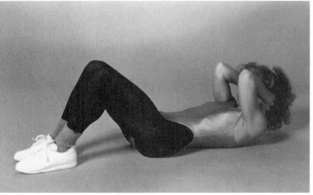

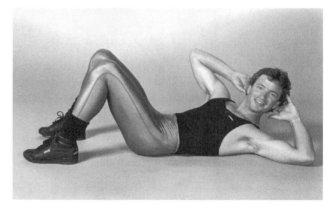

Avoid tucking the chin to the chest.
Avoid bringing elbows up.
Avoid pulling on the neck.

Oblique Curl or Crunch: *targets the* **Internal** *and* **External Obliques.** Lift up leading with shoulder. Bring one elbow to midline of body, resting the opposite elbow on the floor. Keep the chin away from the chest and the elbow back. Exhale as you lift up.

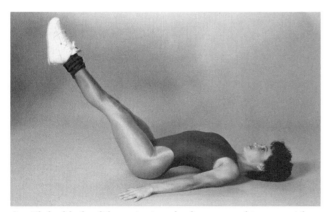

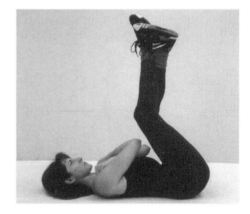

Avoid double leg lifts, swinging the legs, or pushing up with the finger tips.

Reverse Curl: *targets the* **Rectus Abdominus** *and the* **Tranverse Obliques.** Elevate hips off the floor. Keep movements controlled and exhale as you lift up. Careful on the back. Good hamstring flexibility is essential to this exercise's safety.

DON'T

DO

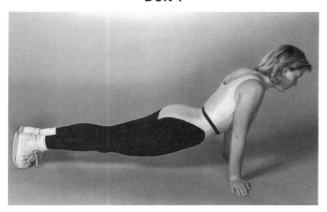

Avoid arching the back. **Avoid** locking the knees or elbows. **Avoid** holding your breath. **Avoid** straining the neck.

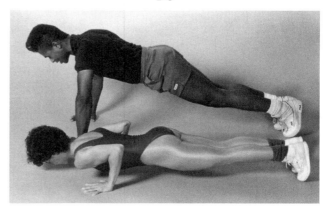

Push-ups: *targets the* **Pectoralis Major and Tripceps.** Start with hands directly below the chest with arms shoulder width apart and elbows slightly bent. Lower the body keeping the head in alignment with the shoulders. Maintain a flat back by contracting the abdominals.

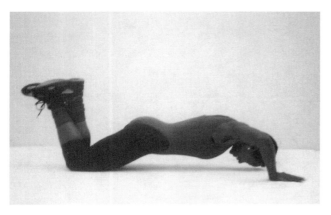

Avoid placing the hands too far forward.
Avoid dropping the head.

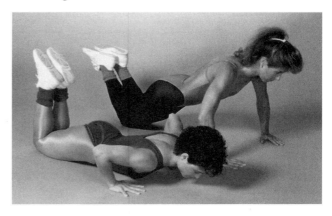

Modified push-ups: *targets the* **Pectoralis Major** *and* **Triceps.** Start with hands directly below the chest with arms shoulder width apart and elbows slightly bent. Lower the body keeping the head in alignment with the shoulders. Maintain a flat black by contracting the abdominals.

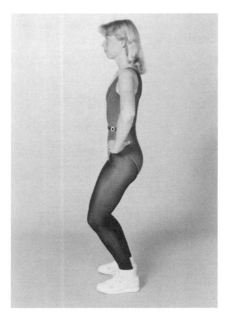

Avoid tucking pelvis under. **Avoid** lifting up with the heels. **Avoid** allowing knees to drop forward.

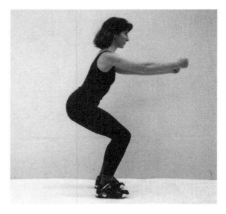

Squats: *targets the* **Quadriceps, Gluteals,** *and* **Hamstrings.** With feet hip distance apart and toes forward or slightly out, lower the body as if sitting in a chair with hips back and knees above the ankle. When returning to the starting position push the heels down.

DON'T

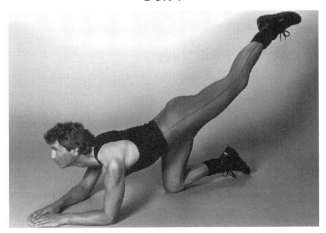

<u>Avoid</u> arching the back. <u>Avoid</u> lifting the head. <u>Avoid</u> lifting the leg above hip level.

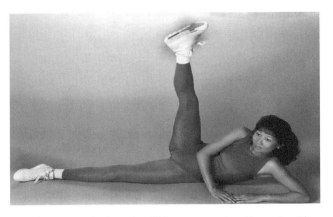

<u>Avoid</u> rotating the hip. <u>Avoid</u> leaning on the elbow. <u>Avoid</u> turning the knee to the ceiling.

DO

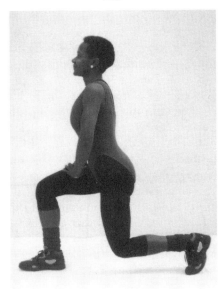

DO

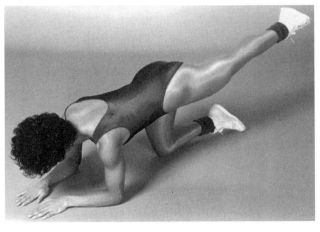

Leg extensions: *targets the* **Gluteals** *and* **Hamstrings.** Distribute body weight equally on both elbows and supporting knee. Contract abdominals and look at the floor. Keep hips even and parallel to the floor. Extend leg until directly in line with the hips. *An optional* **leg curl** *can be performed at the top of the lift by bending the knee and bringing the heel towards the hips.*

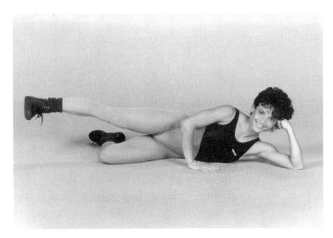

Side leg lift: *targets the* **Abductors** *of the hip.* Bend the bottom leg slightly in front of the body. The upper body is completely on the floor with head resting or supported by the hand. Shoulders and hips are in line. With the toe forward, lift the top leg. *Option: bend both legs at the knee and bring to a 45° in front of the body. Lift the top leg.*

Lunges: *targets the* **Quadriceps, Gluteals,** *and* **Hamstrings.** Stand with feet hip distance apart and one foot in front of the other. Lift the back heel but, keep the front foot on the floor. With weight evenly distributed between both legs, lower the body towards the floor. Keep head up and shoulder back. When returning to the beginning position push down through the front heel. *Option: don't lower the body as far.*

<u>Avoid</u> dropping the chest forward. <u>Avoid</u> lifting up the front heel. <u>Avoid</u> going too low.

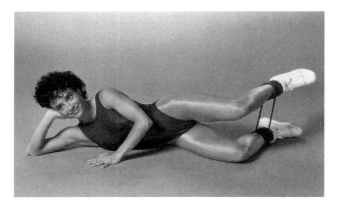

Added resistance using an elastic band.

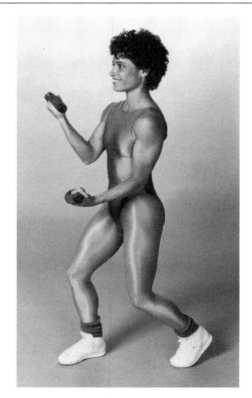

Added resistance using hand weights.

the aerobic segment. Flinging and uncontrolled movements can lead to injury in the upper extremities. All weight resistance exercises should be performed with special consideration to proper alignment and technique.

Many participants try hand weights thinking that they are getting a "better" workout. Using hand weights will elevate heart rate and increase the perception of intensity; however, research shows that minimal increases in cardiovascular benefits result. The bottom line is cardiovascular conditioning is driven by continuous movements of the legs not the arms. Consider the fitness level of an elite cyclist. Bicycling incorporates almost no arm work (other than supporting the upper body), and yet cyclists can achieve maximum training benefits through leg work alone.

Hand weights should not be used to increase the intensity of a workout especially during high impact aerobics. Flinging and uncontrolled movements can lead to injury in the upper extremity. Light hand weights (3 lbs or less) can safely be incorporated during low impact activities when the *goal* is to increase muscular endurance in the upper body. In order to perform this activity safely, music tempo should be lowered, range of motion controlled, and arm work above the head minimized. Basic concerns include maintaining posture, regular breathing and attention to movement variety and alignment.

In a standing position the muscles of the shoulders (deltoids and trapezius) support the arms. Most arm exercises can lead to shoulder fatigue and overuse if movements are not balanced. Structured rest segments should be included during this type of activity and the overall duration limited. Also, any participants with limitations to the shoulder or elbow should not use weights during this activity.

THE FINAL STRETCH AND RELAXATION

The final segment of class should be designed to promote overall flexibility and relax the muscles used during class. Static stretches and controlled breathing are best for accomplishing this. The muscles of the lower body should always be stretched at the end of class with specific attention given to the hamstrings, quadriceps, gastrocnemius, soleus and anterior tibialis. These are the muscles that generate and maintain the movement responsible for cardiovascular conditioning. Upper body stretches should target the specific muscles used during class with additional attention given to stretching the chest and anterior deltoids. These upper body muscles are often tight from daily activities (driving, lifting objects, carrying back packs, etc.), leaving the shoulders rounded and the upper body slightly slouched.

Many students may be anxious to leave early and skip this final portion of the class, so it is necessary to reemphasize the importance of static stretching. Flexibility like any other aspect of fitness can only be developed and maintained through effort. By ignoring flexibility training you will be limiting your own physical potential. Using the initial stretches outlined in Chapter 6 and in

DON'T

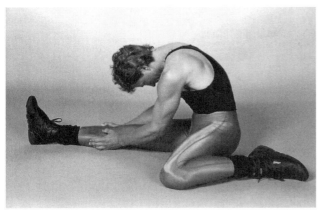

<u>Avoid</u> the hurdler stretch as it places unnecessary stress on the knees.

DO

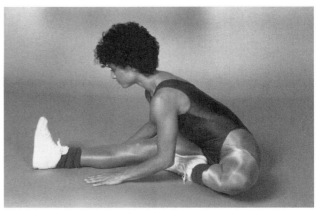

Leg stretch: *targets the* **hamstrings** *individually*. Support the upper body with the hands and lean forward from the hips, not the back.

DON'T

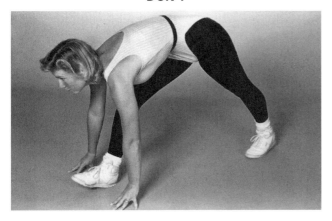

<u>Avoid</u> trying to support the body on the floor while standing. Good posture is sacrificed and stress is placed on the low back.

DO

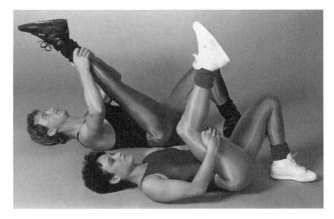

Leg stretch: *targets the* **hamstrings** *individually*. Keep upper body relaxed on the floor. Use the hands to gently bring the leg to the chest. Try to keep the knee straight.

DON'T

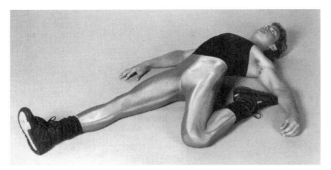

<u>Avoid</u> extreme range of motion. This compromises the back as well as the knee.

DO

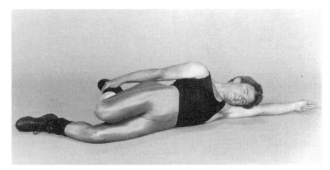

Thigh stretch: *targets the* **quadriceps** *and* **hip flexors.** Lay on the side with the upper body on the ground. Bend the leg at the knee and hold. Grasping the ankle with the hand is optional.

DO

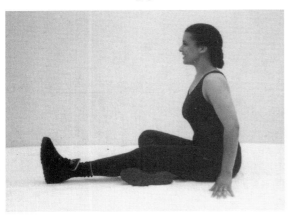

Modify stretches as needed. This hamstring stretch is made easier by placing the bottom leg under the knee.

DO

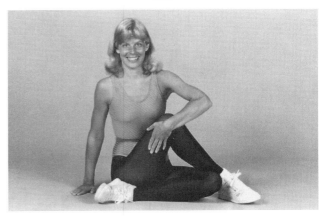

Pretzel stretch: *targets the hip abductors.* Sitting tall bring one foot over the opposite leg near the thigh. Use the hands to gently bring the knee to the chest. Hold this position. *(Option: bottom leg may be straight in front or bent underneath.)*

DO

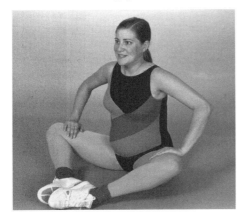

Use gravity and gentle pressure to maximize range of motion. This adductor stretch is challenging because of the relative position and assistance by the hands.

DO

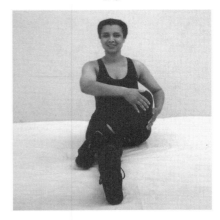

Modify any stretches for comfort and effectiveness. Pictured: **Modified pretzel stretch.**

DO

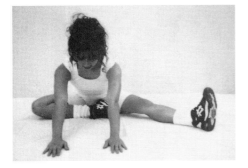

Support the upper body so as to minimize pressure on the back **and to allow muscles to relax.** This modified adductor and hamstring stretch is made more comfortable by using the hands to keep the back straight.

DO

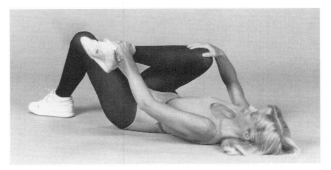

Stretch at your own range of motion. Each of the above stretches targets the hip abductors. The varying positions will change the intensity of the stretch. Not everyone will be able to maintain good posture and hold the pretzel stretch, but most people will be able to try the position on their back.

DON'T

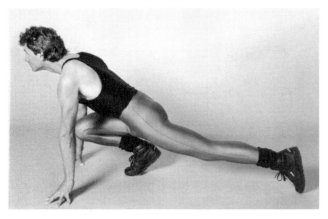

DO

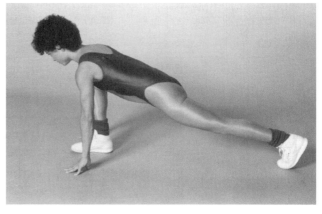

Avoid positions that are too advanced, if you do not have the strength and range of motion to maintain proper alignment.

Try other more challenging positions, but pay attention to technique and body alignment.

DO

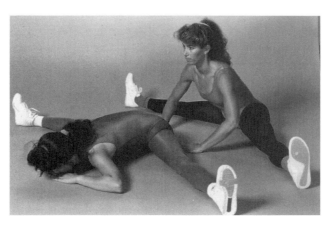

Stretch within your own personal limits.

this chapter, you can maintain and improve your own flexibility by following these specific guidelines:

1. Target the muscles used during the preceding workout or any that feel tense.

2. Increase the range of motion, but still maintain comfortable position.

3. Hold the stretch for 30–60 seconds.

4. During the initial phase of the stretch concentrate on lengthening the muscle and breathing.

5. Take at least ten seconds to emphasize muscle relaxation.

6. To assist with relaxation consciously exhale.

Time always seems to be the limiting factor in post-activity stretching, so additional stretching outside of class is recommended.

SUMMARY

The aerobic cool down, isolated conditioning and final stretch segments are all essential components of a complete aerobic exercise program. No other exercise program can offer such diversity and meet as many physical and mental fitness objectives as a program of this nature. Remember to practice safe and proper exercise techniques to maximize the potential benefits and keep exercise fun and injury free.

HEART RATE	WARM-UP 7–10 MIN.	AEROBIC CONDITIONING 20 MIN. (MINIMUM)	COOL-DOWN 5 MIN.	MUSCULAR ENDURANCE 15–20 MIN.	STRETCHING AND RELAXATION 5 MIN.
200					
190					
180		85%			
170					
160		TRAINING HEART RATE ZONE			
150					
140					
130					
120					
110					
100		60%			
90					
80					
70					
60	BEGIN				END

GLOSSARY

Alignment—refers to body positioning with one segment in line with another.

Cool-Down—the exercise period immediately following the aerobic conditioning segment. The cool-down is designed to reduce the exercise intensity gradually with walking paced rhythmical movements.

Isolated Conditioning—includes a variety of exercises designed to improve muscular strength and endurance. These exercises may be performed standing, sitting or lying on an exercise mat.

Isometric Muscle Contractions—contraction of a muscle for which no movement occurs, e.g., tightening the biceps muscle with the elbow flexed at 90 degrees.

Isotonic Muscle Contraction—contraction of a muscle for which movement occurs, e.g., flexing and extending a body segment.

Recovery Heart Rate—the heart rate taken after the cool-down as a safety indicator that the body has been adequately cooled down. The recovery heart rate should be 120 beats per minute or less (for all participants).

Technique—refers to how a particular movement is performed.

Work gives satisfaction.

—Anne Frank

CHAPTER 10

Variety Training

Cardiovascular conditioning can be derived from a variety of activities; aerobic dance is just one. As you progress in your program, you will develop the endurance to expand your basic workouts. While one way to expand your program is to simply add more days of aerobic dance, exploring and including new activities is strongly recommended. **Variety training** *can prevent boredom and overuse injuries by supplementing a basic aerobic dance program with different cardiovascular activities.* Walking and jumping rope are time honored activities that can be used to supplement an existing cardiovascular program. Water exercise, step aerobics, and sliding are relatively new activities that are also fun to include as individual or group workouts.

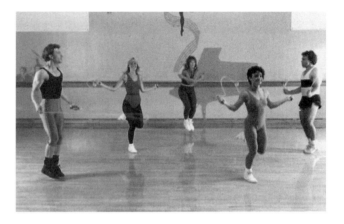

An important concept to understand when developing any new skill is *specificity.* **Specificity** *dictates that activities develop fitness and skill levels independent of each other.* That is, skills and fitness that are developed by participating in a specific activity are not automatically transferred to the performance of another activity. This explains why someone may find swimming one lap exhausting, even if they can run five miles in less than thirty minutes or perform 40 minutes of aerobic dance without fatigue. Specificity is not a limitation but a challenge to develop ourself through new endeavors. So for anyone trying a new skill, be patient. Allow yourself the opportunity to learn without frustration and don't feel compelled to be advanced in terms of skill or intensity. Variety training is a way to broaden your fitness program. The more ways you challenge your body the more ways it has an opportunity to develop.

FITNESS WALKING

Walking for any reason is a recommended part of an active lifestyle. Climbing stairs instead of taking elevators and opting for that parking space not so close to the store are small but important ways we support our fitness. A structured walking program can also provide an enjoyable means of activity for an individual or small group.

Fitness walking is one of the most convenient and assessable physical activities available. The

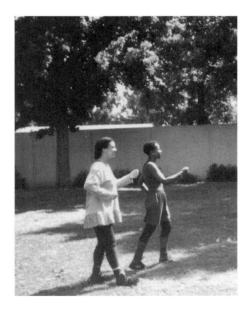

only equipment needed is a good pair of shoes and a little knowledge about technique. **Fitness walking** *incorporates the basic skills of walking combined with enough speed to elevate the heart rate within the training zone.* To increase walking speed you can either increase stride length or take more frequent steps. The latter is recommended and is usually the more comfortable option. Taking larger than normal steps can put extra stress on the back and lower legs, especially when climbing or descending a hill. Taking smaller, more frequent steps makes it easier to maintain proper posture, increase leg speed, and develop the momentum to challenge your heart. The key to fitness walking is to bend the elbows to a 90° angle and then emphasize swinging the arms at the side of the body. Since arms are synchronized with the legs during walking, a rapid arm swing will correspond with faster foot movements. Bending the elbows allows the arms to swing more readily. Even though the arms move quickly, keep the shoulders and hands relaxed. Good posture is upright with the shoulders back. Avoid leaning forward and locking the knees.

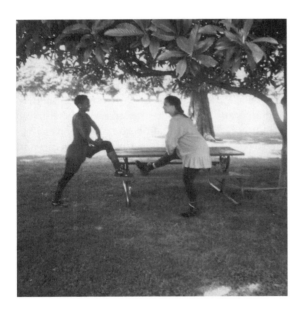

Fitness walking should begin at a slow pace to warm-up the muscles and the speed gradually increased. Fitness walkers also benefit from pre-activity stretches, concentrating on shoulders, back and lower body. During the warm-up, special attention should be given to the shins and calves which are most susceptible to fatigue during walking, espe-cially if on an incline. To minimize tension and promote general flexibility, be sure to stretch after each walking session.

Some people perceive walking as a low intensity activity and incorporate additional resistance, usually hand or ankle weights, in order to increase cardiovascular conditioning. Most fitness experts agree that ankle weights affect normal gait and can lead to knee, back, and joint discomfort. The use of hand or wrist weights is more controversial. However, looking at research and applying what we know about physical conditioning should clarify the issue.

Walking with hand weights tends to elicit higher heart rates and perceived exertion, while oxygen consumption remains about the same. This is consistent with the physical responses of added resistance during other cardiovascular activities. In fact, one study on self-paced walking observed that without hand weights participants walked faster and had greater increases in the aerobic capacity than when resistance was added (Morrow, Bishop, & Teare Ketter, 1992). This is not to dismiss the physical challenge of walking with hand weights, but rather to highlight the possible risks.

The primary concern is overusing the arm and shoulder muscles. As walking incorporates a repetitive arm swing, these muscles are very susceptible to fatigue and strain when resistance is added. This would explain why walking speed may decrease when using hand weights. Also, in the case of arm fatigue, the supporting muscles in the neck and upper back must be recruited to sustain movement. Tension in these muscles affect normal posture and can also lead to added discomfort and strain. Using hand weights should be done with discretion and only by trained individuals. Limit resistance to one half or pound. Remember the key to fitness walking is maintaining a challenging pace. Additional intensity can also be achieved by climbing and descending hills.

Effective fitness walking should include comfortable shoes appropriate for the activity. Walking shoes are distinct from aerobic shoes. Walking, like running, incorporates a repetitive foot pattern where the heel strikes the ground first. Because there is less impact during walking than jogging a pair of inexpensive running shoes are very effective for most walking activities. Cross-trainers can also be used by many walking enthusiasts. For hiking over uneven terrain, shoes with additional support is recommended.

JUMPING ROPE

Jumping rope is a very challenging activity that can be used to supplement an existing fitness program. For adults, jumping rope is best done in training intervals. That is, short sessions of jumping followed by intervals of walking, marching in place, or other less intense activity. Table 10-1 lists sample sessions based on fitness level. Progression through these intervals will take time and practice. Hopping and skipping either forward or backwards are all skills that can be incorporated at any level of training. When first beginning, use the skills that are the easiest for you. This will give you the best opportunity to practice and assist you in progressing to the next level of training.

Jumping rope *is a high intensity and high-impact cardiovascular exercise.* An interval format will help keep the activity from being too intense. You may choose to do a total of five or ten minutes of jumping intervals followed by another activity. This is especially effective for peaking a workout. Because of the intensity of this activity, a complete warm-up and cool down is very important. Jumping rope should be performed on a quality surface with a good pair of shoes. Aerobic footwear or quality cross trainers will likely work best. Good technique includes bending the knees with each step, landing using the entire foot, and controlled arm movements. To protect the arm and shoulders swing the rope using initially the forearm and maintain the movement with the wrist.

WATER EXERCISE

Swimming is the traditional water activity for promoting cardiovascular fitness. Swimming is an individual exercise where the body is suspended and propelled through water. Water exercise is an alternative form of training that can also be performed in the pool. **Water exercise** *is distinct from swimming and generally consists of movements performed to music while standing in shallow water or using floatation devices in the deep end of the pool.* This activity can also be performed in groups, adding a social aspect to the exercising in the pool. Strong swimming skills are not necessary, but water exercise participants must feel comfortable in the water and should be supervised by qualified personnel if they do not swim.

Water is an effective exercise medium, providing a cool, low-impact and resistive environment. Depending on the facility being used, pool temperatures will vary between 78–86°. This will keep the

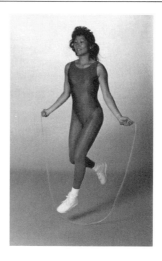

TABLE 10-1		
Intervals		
	Jumping rope	Walking
Beginning activity	15 seconds	45 seconds
	20–30 seconds	30–40 seconds
	45 seconds	30 seconds
Advanced activity	60 seconds	30 seconds

body cool during exercise and minimize the sense of fatigue or exhaustion. When exercising in the pool the effect of gravity is decreased. If the body is submerged to approximately chest level, jogging or walking on the pool bottom is a low-impact activity that can be enjoyed by a variety of exercise enthusiasts. If suspended in deep water using flotation devices, water exercise provides a non-impact yet challenging workout.

Water also provides multi-dimensional resistance and support. While bending and extending the leg, water resists the movement in each direction and provides an effective and balanced means for building muscular strength and endurance. More resistance is encountered when the arms and legs are fully extended and less when the knees and elbows are bent. Increasing the surface area of the feet and hands provides additional resistance. This can be achieved by using shoes and gloves or by simply cupping the hands during movement. The same property in water that provides resistance also supports the body. This support, when coupled with the low-impact nature of water exercise, provides a safe and comfortable environment for individuals with back discomfort and other muscular-skeletal concerns.

TABLE 10-2

Tips for Exercising in the Water

To Keep Warm

cover exposed skin to trap body heat by

1. wearing a cap to cover the head
2. wearing a close fitting t-shirt

To Increase the Resistance

increase the surface area in the direction of the movement by

1. keeping arms and legs extended but knees and elbows slightly bent
2. cupping the hands
3. occasionally pointing the toes during movements (constant pointing of the toes may cause cramping in the lower leg)
4. wearing gloves and shoes
5. traveling forward or backward

To Decrease the Resistance

decrease the surface area in the direction of the movement by

1. bending the knees and elbows during movement
2. slicing the hands through the water
3. keeping the foot flexed during movements
4. remaining in place or traveling sideways

Water exercise is a safe and effective activity for most people; however, good technique is still important. Keeping the knees and elbows slightly bent protects the joints from the extra resistance. The trunk should be used to stabilize the body in the water allowing the arms and legs to perform the movements. Arms should be used under the water and movements that bring the arms in and out of the water should be avoided unless actually swimming. When using flotation devices incorporate a variety of arm positions in order to avoid upper body fatigue. Like traditional aerobics, movement speed during water exercise is not the key to intensity, but rather continuous activity through a controlled range of motion. Table 10-2 includes some tips that will help personalize water exercise.

SLIDING

Sliding incorporates movements reminiscent of cross country skiing and in-line skating. **Sliding** *is a low impact activity involving lateral movements performed on a specialized sliding board.* To minimize friction, the surface of a sliding board is slick and booties are worn over shoes, allowing the foot to glide easily over the surface. Moving back and forth to music, sliding can incorporate slow gliding movements, sliding and lifting, or quick shuffling in place. Many slide boards have adjustable lengths allowing beginners practice and develop endurance, using smaller movements. Once skills and endurance have been developed, the board can be adjusted so longer strides can be taken.

Safe sliding incorporates a strong body position from the feet to the arms. Smooth, continuous gliding is impossible without muscular control and the appropriate amount of foot pressure applied to the board. The knees must remain slightly bent throughout each stride. In order to maintain a neutral spine position, a forward body lean must be initiated from the hips and not the low back. Participants must be sure to <u>warm up the knees and legs rhythmically in place before performing lateral sliding movements.</u> After each slide session, be sure to stretch the hip abductors and adductors.

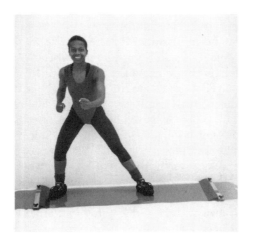
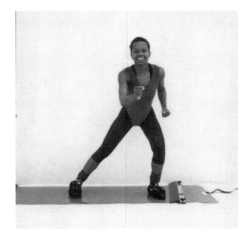

STEP AEROBICS

Remember when you were told (ordered) to run the stadium stairs? For many students such instructions were accompanied a feeling of dread. Well, the activity of stair climbing has been elevated to new heights. Still just as challenging but no longer feared, stepping up and down on platforms is the popularized version of climbing stadium stairs. No, this is not really new, but students often think so. This modern version of stair climbing can incorporate a variety of movements and can be used to develop aerobic capacity, coordination, or muscular strength and endurance.

Step aerobics *is a cardiovascular activity where the body moves vertically up and down on a bench or platform.* Like aerobic dance, intensity is generated by the vertical movement of the body's center of gravity. Lifting the body repeatedly up and down requires strong leg movements, providing effective lower body toning in addition to cardiovascular training. Step aerobics provides movement options that basic stair climbing cannot. The step platform allows for movements in a variety of directions. Basic movement options include approaching the step from the front, side, end, top or even straddled. From there, movements become quite diverse. There are many brands of step platforms with varying dimensions and features. In accommodating different skill and fitness levels, platforms that have

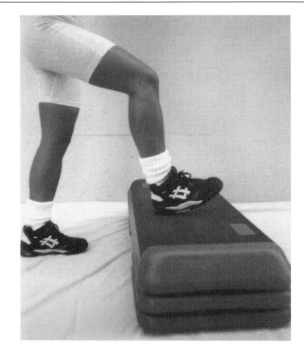

adjustable heights provide the most versatility for physical needs.

Typically, platforms will vary from four, six, and eight inches. A participant new to step activities should begin with the lowest level, even if they are already active in an aerobic program. Step movements are quite unique and may take time to

TABLE 10-3	
Recommended Stepping Technique	
Things To Do	**Things Not To Do**
1. Pick a platform height based on *LEG LENGTH, FITNESS & SKILL LEVEL*	1. Avoid flexing the knees beyond 90° when weight bearing: select the appropriate platform height
2. Keep movements controlled by using step music approximately 120–125 bpm	2. Avoid uncontrolled movements especially when executing turns and directional changes
3. When stepping up, place the entire foot on the platform, landing heel first	3. Avoid landing toe first or allowing the heels to hang off the rear of the platform
4. Always keep the shoulders back and relaxed, chest up, back neutral, and knees bent	4. Avoid bending from waist or arching the back, especially when stepping up
5. When stepping down, bend the knees and roll from the ball of the foot to the heel	5. Avoid locking the knees and remaining on the toes when stepping down
6. Use a variety of movement combinations, limiting repetitions on each leg	6. Avoid overusing the hip flexors (extension, abduction, & adduction are part of a balanced workout)
7. Lift/move the platform by using the legs	7. Avoid lifting or moving the platform with the back

Adapted from Francis, L., Francis, P. & Miller, G. (1990). *Step Reebok Training Manual.* Stoughton, MA: Reebok International Ltd.

master safely. Using the lowest bench height will provide the greatest success. After students have developed the basic skills they can change the height of their platform. The class level, music speed, movement complexity, and individual leg length are all considerations for choosing the appropriate step height. While the other condi-

tions may vary from class to class, the overall step height should not cause the knee to bend beyond 90°, as this puts unnecessary strain on the joint.

In evaluating step aerobics, initial research indicates that step movements are relatively low-impact when one foot remains in contact with the step (Francis & Francis, 1990; Francis, 1993). **Propulsion** *is a step technique that incorporates a small controlled hop on top of the platform and can be used to increase intensity.* Propulsion can be safely used by most participants but with the understanding that it will increase the impact of the activity. Propulsion on the step is an effective way to increase with intensity without raising the platform, but hops should be executed with control and at the discretion of the participant.

Step classes are very popular throughout the country but vary in both content and execution. Some classes can be very basic, involving simple steps and lifts. Other classes can be very intricate, involving propulsion and turns that require more strength and skill. It is important to participate in a class that is appropriate to your skill level and elicits no physical discomfort. Individuals with knee concerns should take step classes with discretion, especially in terms of step height and lateral movements. Study table 10-3 and the technique described in the following pictures to learn more about safe stepping.

DON'T

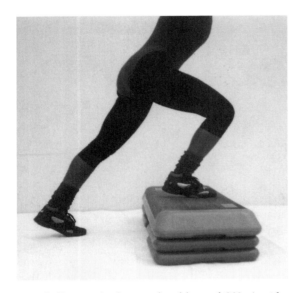

Avoid allowing the knee to bend beyond 90°. **Avoid** stepping too far behind the platform. **Avoid** leaning too far forward.

DON'T

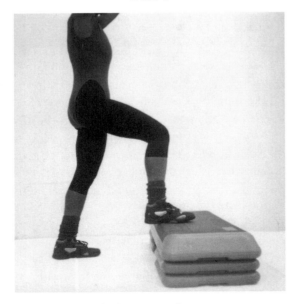

Avoid placing only the toes on the step.

DO

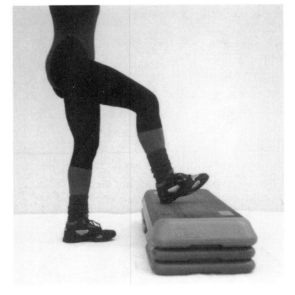

Land with the heel first, placing the entire foot on the platform. Keep the knee above the ankle.

DON'T

DO

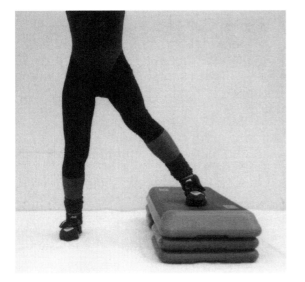

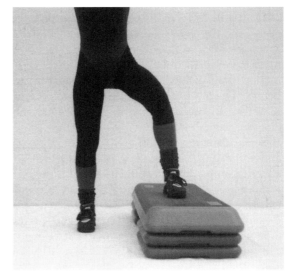

Avoid rotating the knee inward as this will put pressure on the joint.

Keep the knees in line with the feet.

DO

DO

DO

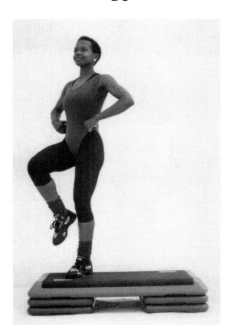

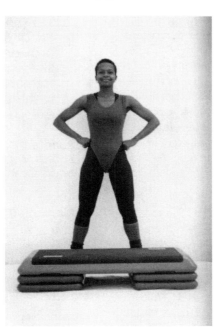

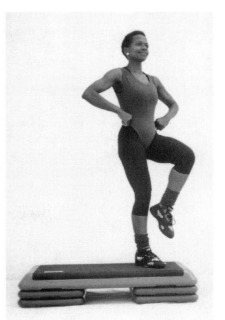

When traveling corner to corner, land with feet apart on the floor. This will minimize twisting of the knees.

OTHER ACTIVITIES

Many other activities can be used to promote fitness and cardiovascular conditioning. **Tai chi** is a popular form of martial arts that involves fluid movements performed in a controlled range of motion. It is a low-impact activity that has the potential to develop balance, agility, coordination, as well as, strength, endurance, flexibility and cardiovascular function.

Social dancing is another way to promote an active lifestyle. Country line dancing, ballroom dancing, and many cultural dances are being performed around the country. These are fun and effective ways to both socialize and remain active. To help you learn general movements and specific dance patterns, lessons are available usually through a local college, recreation facility, or night club.

Sport and recreational skills are an important part of an active lifestyle and, depending on the nature of the activity, can also be used to promote aerobic endurance. While golf, sailing, and fishing make only limited contributions to cardiovascular conditioning, soccer, tennis, and basketball all have the potential to significantly improve fitness.

Traditional aerobic activities use rhythmical and continuous movements of the legs. Cardiovascular conditioning is also recommended to maintain a moderate intensity. In the strictest definitions many sport skills may not appear to be aerobic in nature, but research indicates benefits do exist. Basketball, for example, incorporates sprinting, jogging, walking and standing at a moments notice. In a game situation, most sports do not provide continuous movement nor a consistent intensity. However, with these and other intermittent activities the heart is challenged, even if only for a short period of time.

GUIDELINES FOR ACTIVITY SELECTION

Activity selection is really a matter of personal choice. The following considerations may help you find the activities best suited to your needs.

- **IMPACT:** Some activities, jumping rope, traditional aerobics, and running involve impact forces several times your body weight. Skills that are less jarring include water exercise, walking, or step aerobics.
- **CONVENIENCE:** Many activities are dependent on weather, access to a health club, or expensive equipment. Try activities that you can easily perform year-round.
- **SKILL:** Some activities such as step aerobics, aerobic dance, and rope jumping require more time and practice to master. Allow time for these skills to develop.
- **ENJOYMENT:** Activities that provide enjoyment are more likely to be continued. The training effect of exercise will result only from regular exercise.

Adapted from American College of Sports Medicine (1992). *ACSM fitness book*. Champaign, IL: Leisure Press.

SUMMARY

Variety training is a safe and effective way to supplement an exercise program. Incorporating a different activity builds new skills, assists ongoing motivation, and contributes to overall fitness. Exercise specificity means that each new activity should be approached as a learning experience. Walking, jumping rope, stepping, sliding and water aerobics are all effective ways to improve cardiovascular fitness. These activities can be performed individually or with a group. The key to a successful and fun program is to explore your exercise options.

GLOSSARY

Fitness Walking—incorporates the basic skills of walking combined with enough speed to elevate the heart rate within the training zone.

Jumping Rope—a high intensity and high impact activity cardiovascular exercise.

Mall Walking—fitness walking performed inside shopping malls; a weather proof, climate controlled social activity that can be performed year round.

Propulsion—small controlled hop performed on

top of the step platform; generally safe movements for most participants but will increase the impact of the activity.

Sliding—a low impact activity involving lateral, gliding movements performed on a specialized sliding board.

Specificity—dictates that fitness and skills developed through one activity are independent and not transferred to other activities without practice.

Step Aerobics—a cardiovascular activity where the body moves vertically up and down on a platform.

Variety Training—can prevent boredom and overuse injuries by supplementing a basic aerobic dance program with different cardiovascular activities.

Water Exercise—movements generally performed to music while standing in shallow water or using flotation devices in deep water; pool exercises distinct from swimming.

REFERENCES

Armstrong, N. (1987). Walking: Fitness afoot. Diabetes Forecast, 302. (A publication of the American Diabetes Association, P.O. Box 2043, Mahopac, NY 10541).

Francis, L. (1993). Teaching Step Training. *Journal of Health Physical Education Recreation and Dance*, March, 26–30.

Francis, L., Francis, P. & Miller, G. (1990). *Step Reebok Training Manual*. Stoughton, MA: Reebok International Ltd.

Kravitz, L. & Deivert, R. (1991). The safe way to stepping. *Dance Exercise Today*, 9 (4), 47–50.

Morrow, S. K., Bishop, & Teare Ketter, C. A. (1992). Energy cost of self-paced walking with handheld weights. *Research Quarterly for Exercise and Sport*, 63 (4), 435–437.

Sova, R. (1991). *Aquatics*. Boston: Jones and Bartlett Publishers.

CHAPTER 11

General Nutrition

Proper nutrition, a balanced diet and regular exercise are essential for good physical and mental health. You will not be able to establish nor sustain an active lifestyle without the support of the nutrients that provide your body with energy and regulate your metabolism. Not only does eating well necessitate planning and preparation, it requires dedication and a lifelong commitment to wellness. This chapter describes the fundamental principles of nutrition to guide you further in your quest for a healthier and happier life.

THE SCIENCE OF NUTRITION

Nutrition is the study of the foods we consume and the mechanisms by which these foods are metabolized by the body. Foods supply us with the nutrients essential for building and repairing the body tissues. They also provide the energy needed for efficient functioning. You are probably familiar with the principles of basic nutrition that were taught to you in school and at home. Still, knowing and understanding does little good unless you use those principles to make proper nutrition a lifetime habit that you take the time to practice every day. Poor nutritional habits have been linked to numerous systemic illnesses and disease, not to mention obesity. Proper nutrition and regular exercise work well together to prevent a variety of disorders and control body weight. To fully appreciate weight management and the inter-relationship between exercise and diet you must first understand basic nutrition.

THE ROLE OF ESSENTIAL NUTRIENTS IN BODY FUNCTION

Nutrients consists of elements and compounds found in the foods we eat. There are **six essential nutrients:** carbohydrates, protein, fats, vitamins, minerals, and water. The term "essential" means that the body cannot function normally without certain nutrients. Daily intake of the essential nutrients is recommended because they are not manufactured in the body and are stored/available only in limited quantities. The first three nutrients (carbohydrates, protein, and fats) each contain calories which, when broken down through chemical processes, provide energy to individual cells. Any excess calories not used to provide energy or used for other essential body functions are stored as fat in **adipose tissue.** This is true whether those excess calories were initially from fat, protein or carbohydrates. Vitamins and minerals are necessary to help regulate the chemical processes that convert calories into usable energy but contain no calories themselves. Water is necessary to maintain fluid balance, thus assisting in regulating blood volume, body temperature, and the proper functioning of the kidneys.

Carbohydrates

The primary function of carbohydrates is to provide the body with a continuous supply of energy. **Carbohydrates** *are the preferred fuel of nervous tissue, and assist in digestion, help to regulate protein and fat metabolism, and are required for the breakdown of fat within the liver.* They also provide the energy needed to sustain basic body function as well as recreational activity. Carbohydrates are derived primarily from plants and are present in foods in the form of sugars, starches and cellulose. The simple sugars (fruits and honey) are easily digested and immediately metabolized for quick energy. The double sugars (table sugar) require slightly more digestive action to be metabolized. The complex sugars or starches (grains, cereals, pasta, bread) require an even greater enzymatic action to be broken down and metabolized for energy. This means that more

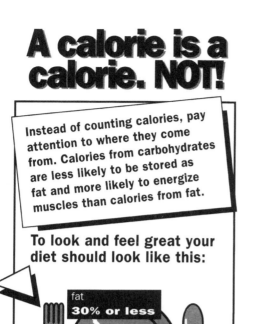

A calorie is a calorie. NOT!

Instead of counting calories, pay attention to where they come from. Calories from carbohydrates are less likely to be stored as fat and more likely to energize muscles than calories from fat.

To look and feel great your diet should look like this:

fat
30% or less

carbohydrates
55-60%

protein
10-15%

Less means more!

Bite for bite, complex carbs like those found in grain foods contain less than half the calories found in fat.

1 fat gram

equals 9 calories

1 carbohydrate gram

equals 4 calories

There's no need to starve! If you fill up on high-carb foods you can eat more and have less to burn off at the gym and more energy to build muscle. That's why dietary guidelines recommend 6 to 11 servings of carbohydrate-rich grain foods such as bread, cereal, pasta, crackers and rice.

calories are used in the energy making process. Carbohydrates are also a source of dietary fiber. Fiber such as cellulose (found in wheat products) and pectin (fruit and vegetable skins) is not digestible by humans, but instead assists in intestinal motility and the elimination of waste.

All carbohydrates, with the exception of fiber, are broken down into simple sugars (glucose) before they are transferred to each cell and used for energy. Once the capacity of the cell has been reached, some of the glucose is converted to glycogen and stored in the liver and muscles for later use. Any excess carbohydrates that cannot be stored are then converted to fat, sent to the various adipose sites around the body, and maintained as a reserve energy supply. This explains why a person eating a low fat and moderate protein diet might gain weight if their caloric intake exceeds their body's need for nutrients. Only when the adipose reserves are broken down into usable components and metabolized will fat weight loss result.

A diet high in simple sugars but low in starches creates a nutritional deficit. Over indulgence like this can lead to weight gain. Obesity is directly related to coronary heart disease, the onset of diabetes, kidney disorders and cancer.

Is a low carbohydrate diet the way to lose weight? Definitely not. The stores of carbohydrates in the muscles and liver are limited. Your body needs carbohydrates, especially complex sugars, to maintain normal function everyday. Did you know that your brain prefers carbohydrates as a source of energy? Remember the last time you skipped a meal or fasted. Were you tired; unable to concentrate? Did you experience a dull headache? That was your brains way of saying it needs more carbohydrates. The average brain requires approximately 600 calories from carbohydrates each day. Can you see how fasting and inadequate carbohydrate intake would affect your ability to function efficiently. As a result of a low carbohydrate diet or fasting, your body must seek out other less efficient forms of energy to sustain body function. If you engage in vigorous physical activity and maintain a low carbohydrate diet (little or no glycogen on reserve) your body will eventually break down protein for energy. Muscle protein is often sacrificed during this process. The fat stores are left largely untouched because your body's protective mechanism, which reserves fat for last resort energy, does not know if you are starving yourself or simply on a diet. Meanwhile, as muscle protein is used for energy, lean body mass (muscle) is lost instead of fat.

Americans consume about 50% of their diet in carbohydrates. Unfortunately, the complex carbohydrates constitute only a small portion of this. The recommended daily intake of carbohydrates is between 55 and 65% of the total diet, with the majority of calories coming from complex sugars. Take a look at your diet. Are you eating a variety of complex carbohydrates? Is your daily intake of

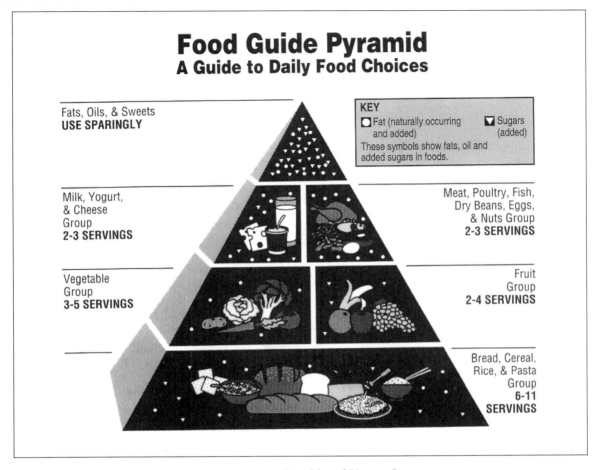

Food Guide Pyramid
A Guide to Daily Food Choices

Fats, Oils, & Sweets
USE SPARINGLY

KEY
☐ Fat (naturally occurring and added)   ▼ Sugars (added)
These symbols show fats, oil and added sugars in foods.

Milk, Yogurt, & Cheese Group
2-3 SERVINGS

Meat, Poultry, Fish, Dry Beans, Eggs, & Nuts Group
2-3 SERVINGS

Vegetable Group
3-5 SERVINGS

Fruit Group
2-4 SERVINGS

Bread, Cereal, Rice, & Pasta Group
6-11 SERVINGS

Source: U.S. Department of Agriculture/Department of Health and Human Services.

simple carbohydrates too high? By evaluating your diet, you can better understand how your total body weight, body composition and nutritional state are affected.

Fats

Fats have several key functions in the body. During an aerobic state, a gram of fat yields twice as much energy as a gram of carbohydrates. The *primary function of* **fat** *is to provide a continuous supply of energy to the body*. In addition, fats transport fat soluble vitamins (A, D, E, & K), and assist in the absorption of vitamin D, making calcium available to strengthen bones, teeth, and body tissues. Fats also protect vital organs and provide insulation to resist cold.

Fats come from the plants and animal products we eat. The dietary fats we eat are called triglycerides. Broken down each triglyceride yields three fatty acid chains and a glycerol molecule. Fatty acids circulate through the blood stream and are used for energy by the muscles. The body simulta-

TABLE 11-1
Reading Your Ingredient List.

The first item on an ingredient list is the primary element found in that food. Each other item is listed in descending order. So a food will be high in sugar if the first item listed is a sugar or if several sugars are listed on label.

Sugars by other Names:

sucrose (table sugar)	honey
brown sugar	syrup
raw sugar	corn sweetener
glucose (dextrose)	high-fructose
fructose	corn syrup
maltose	molasses
lactose	fruit juice concentrate

Adapted from the U.S. Department of Agriculture and the U.S. Department of Health and Human Services, 1990, third edition.

neously burns carbohydrates (glucose) and fat (fatty acids) during both rest and activity. However, the body prefers to use fat as a fuel for muscular function during aerobic activities. At rest the need for calories are relatively few, so the number of fatty acids consumed is minimal. In contrast, during sustained, moderate level cardiovascular activity, when caloric requirements are relatively high, the body has the potential to shift calorie consumption to fatty acids while glucose use is limited.

There are two basic types of fatty acids: saturated and unsaturated. Saturated fats come from animal products and are characteristically solid at room temperature. Unsaturated fatty acids are derived from plant products and in their natural state are liquid at room temperature. Some fatty acids can be manufactured in the body but other, "essential fatty acids", must be ingested in the food we eat. Thirty grams of unsaturated oil will meet the body's requirements for the essential fatty acids. However, most Americans far exceed the minimum daily requirement of fat.

Something most of us know is that fat tastes good. Whether you like butter, ice cream, mayonnaise, prime ribs, or avocados chances are that we like or even crave several foods that are high in fat. Well, you're not alone. Estimations tell us that Americans consume liberal amounts of fatty food and that fat makes up as much as 40–50% of the American diet. Many experts feel this is one of the contributing factors to the high death rate from CHD (Coronary Heart Disease). Three of the primary risk factors for coronary heart disease, obesity, cholesterol levels, and high blood pressure can be linked to diet and more specifically to a high consumption of saturated fat.

Unfortunately, a large percentage of this intake is made up of the saturated fats and cholesterol. Together, these fats are capable of producing very high blood fat levels. An excessive amount of saturated fats in the blood stream have been directly linked to coronary heart disease, arteriosclerosis (building up of plaque on the artery walls), colon cancer and stomach cancer. Nutritionists suggest that an intake of fat which provides 25–30% of the total daily caloric consumption is compatible with good health. They also recommended that a large portion of the fats come from the unsaturated group (vegetable oils).

While a fat deficiency is not likely to occur, a diet containing too little fat may produce a vitamin deficiency in any of the fat soluble vitamins, A, D, E and/or K. Self-induced starvation such as anorexia nervosa or bulimia, can result in serious illness or even death as a consequence of too little dietary fat. Both of these conditions have serious health implications and should be referred for medical attention.

Protein

Protein is found in plants (cereals and grains) and animal products (meat, fish, poultry, eggs, and dairy). Among its numerous functions, **protein** *provides the building materials for the skin, hair, nails, bones, muscles, internal organs, blood and enzymes. Protein is made of small chemical chains called* **amino acids.** Amino acids are the actual building material found in protein. Some amino acids can be synthesized or manufactured in the body, while other "essential amino acids" must be provided by the diet.

Not every source of protein can provide all the essential amino acids. *Animal products contain all the essential amino acids and are considered a* **"complete protein".** However, *all plant protein lacks one or more essential amino acid rendering it an* **"incomplete protein".** This is an important consideration for **vegetarians** *who minimize eating animal products* or **vegans who** *include only plant products.* In order to ensure that all essential amino acids are provided through their food, vegan and vegetarians need to combine plant proteins. Practically, this means eating a variety of grains and legumes together such as beans and rice or bread and peanut butter. Careful menu planning is essential to good health.

While some individuals need to be concerned with consuming enough complete protein, most Americans have the opposite concern. The average American eats more protein than their body requires. Protein should comprise only 10–12% of the total calories consumed each day. The human body circulates only a limited supply of amino acids in the blood stream which can be taken in by cells and used for building. Some amino acids are stored in the liver, but any excess amino acids are converted to fat and stored in adipose tissue.

Protein does supply the body with calories; however, amino acids serve more important body functions than as a source of energy. When the carbohydrate supply in the diet is insufficient the body will break down protein for energy. This explains how muscle tissue is sacrificed during fasting or when on a low carbohydrate diet.

The body works very efficiently, using only what it needs. Unfortunately, too much protein can also make a person fat. Excess calories in the diet, regardless of the source (carbohydrates, fats, protein), can also contribute to an overfat condition. It is best to avoid overindulgence altogether.

Overindulgence is likely to be more common than a diet containing too little protein, except among persons with eating disorders. A low protein diet can lead to abnormal growth and tissue development with a subsequent loss in muscle tone. Hair, skin, and nails are affected immediately when a diet lacks protein. Hair looses its luster and shine, becoming dull and dry. The skin loses its natural glow and is subject to acne. The nails can become weak and fail to grow as quickly as they should. Persons with a protein deficiency may display a general lack of vigor, followed by depression, weakness and a low resistance to infection with a possible delay in the normal recovery process.

Water

Water is the last of the essential nutrients for life, but certainly not the least. The human body is made up of 60–80% liquid of which 40–60% is water. Water is supplied to the body through various fluids and foods (mostly fruits and vegetables) and lost through evaporation, excretion and expiration processes. Unfortunately, it is the most overlooked of the essential nutrients. Our desire for water is largely maintained by the thirst mechanism. But, in reality, the thirst mechanism is a sign of need after the fact. Proper hydration is essential to life and particularly necessary for the exercising individual. During vigorous exercise, the loss of body fluids begins to compromise the body's ability to regulate its core temperature. This places an additional stress on the cardiovascular system. As dehydration continues the heart rate increases, causing less blood to circulate to the skin because less blood enters the heart between beats. As a result, the exercise activity becomes uncomfortable and difficult. An exercise participant may even suffer from heat exhaustion or in extreme cases, heat stroke.

Proper hydration is essential to good performance. A minimum of eight glasses of water a day, with two to three glasses about two to three hours prior to exercise, should serve to adequately hydrate the individual. Water should be consumed as many times as desired during the exercise activity. Remember, water will help to keep you cool. So drink plenty of it!

Vitamins

For the body to maintain basic life processes, all of the nutrients must be adequately present within the diet. **Vitamins** *have no caloric value but function as catalysts in almost all metabolic reactions, regulating*

TABLE 11-2

Nutrient	% of Recommended Daily Intake for Adults (excluding pregnant and lactating women)
	Percent of your daily calories
PROTEIN	10–20%
CARBOHYDRATES	50–55%
simple carbohydrates	< 10%
FATS	< 30%
saturated	< 10%

metabolic processes, converting fat and carbohydrates to energy and assisting in the formation of bones and tissues. There are numerous vitamins present in varying amounts in many foods, all of which are essential for growth and health maintenance. With the exception of a few vitamins, the body cannot synthesize them and must seek supplements through the diet. For women it is very important that their diet is rich in calcium. Calcium is essential for maintaining bone density. Diets low in calcium have been linked to osteoporosis. Dairy products are good sources of calcium, but many people are allergic to them. For individuals who are lactose intolerant, alternative sources of calcium can be found in broccoli, bok choy, sardines, legumes, and may need to seek supplementation. Also, calcium supplementation may play an assistive role in regulating blood pressure of individuals who are hypertensive (Kristal-Boneh & Green, 1992).

Minerals

Minerals are also essential to the life process. *Primarily they assist in the maintenance of normal physiological and musculoskeletal function.* Minerals act as catalysts in numerous biologic functions including the nervous system, digestive system, and the process of nutrient utilization as derived from food stuffs. Minerals help to regulate the body's pH balance and take part in the production of various hormones. All minerals must be supplied through the diet, which means that the body relies upon well balanced meals to maintain normal health. Many diets are lacking in iron. Iron serves the important function in blood of helping oxygen molecules bind to hemoglobin. Iron deficiencies can lead to anemia, a condition characterized by

TABLE 11-3
Summary of the Water-Soluble Vitamins, Their Functions, Deficiency Conditions, and Food Sources

Vitamin	Major Functions	Deficiency Symptoms	Dietary Sources	RDA
Thiamin	Energy metabolism; nerve function	Beriberi; poor coordination, edema, weakness	Sunflower seeds, pork, whole and enriched grains, dried beans, peas, brewers yeast	1.1–1.5 milligrams
Riboflavin	Energy metabolism	Inflammation of mouth and tongue, cracks at corners of the mouth, eye disorders	Milk, mushrooms, spinach, liver, enriched grains	1.2–1.7 milligrams
Niacin	Energy metabolism, fat breakdown	Pellagra; diarrhea	Mushrooms, bran, tuna, salmon, chicken, beef, liver, peanuts, enriched grains	15–19 milligrams
Pantothenic acid	Fat synthesis, fat breakdown	Tingling in hands, fatigue, headache, nausea	Mushrooms, liver, broccoli, eggs; most foods have some	4–7 milligrams
Biotin	Glucose production; fat synthesis	Dermatitis, tongue soreness, anemia, depression	Cheese, egg yolks, cauliflower, peanut butter, liver	30–100 micrograms
Vitamin B-6	Protein metabolism; related to red blood cell synthesis	Headache, anemia, convulsions, nausea, vomiting, flaky skin, sore tongue	Animal protein foods, spinach, broccoli, bananas, salmon, sunflower seeds	1.8–2 milligrams
Folate (folic acid)	DNA and RNA synthesis; amino acid synthesis	Anemia, inflammation of tongue, diarrhea, poor growth	Green leafy vegetables, orange juice, organ meats, sprouts, sunflower seeds	180–200 micrograms
Vitamin B-12	Nerve function	Anemia, poor nerve function	Animal foods, especially organ meats, oysters, clams (not natural in plants)	2 micrograms
Vitamin C	Collagen synthesis; hormone synthesis	Scurvy; poor wound healing, bleeding gums	Citrus fruits, strawberries, broccoli, greens	60 milligrams

continued on next page

TABLE 11-3 (continued)
Summary of the Fat-Soluble Vitamins, Their Functions, Deficiency Conditions, and Food Sources

Vitamin	Major Functions	Deficiency Symptoms	Dietary Sources	RDA
Vitamin A (Beta carotene)	Vision, light and color Promote growth Prevent drying of skin and eyes Promote resistance to bacterial infection	Night blindness Poor growth Dry skin	Vitamin A Liver Fortified milk Beta carotene Sweet potatoes Spinach Greens Carrots Cantaloupe Apricots Broccoli	Females: 800 RE* (4000 IU†) Males: 1000 RE* (5000 IU†)
Vitamin D	Increases absorption of calcium and phosphorus Maintain optimum calcification of bone	Rickets Bone malformation	Vitamin D-fortified milk Fish oils Tuna fish Salmon	5–10 micrograms (200–400 IU)
Vitamin E	Antioxidant: prevent breakdown of vitamin A	Hemolysis of red blood cells Nerve destruction	Vegetable oils Some greens Some fruits	Females: 8 milligrams Males: 10 milligrams
Vitamin K	Helps form blood clotting agents	Abnormal blood clotting	Green vegetables Liver	60–80 micrograms

*Retinol equivalents.
†International units.
Adapted from Wardlaw, G. M. & Insel, P. M. (1993). *Perspectives in Nutrition* (2nd ed.). St. Louis: Mosby.

a low red blood cell count. Foods rich in iron include spinach, raisins, and oysters.

The question regarding the need to supplement the diet with vitamins and/or minerals is best answered by a nutrition expert. There are, however, several recommendations that apply specifically to females. Research has shown repeatedly that many women are not getting enough calcium or iron in the diet. Deficiencies in calcium are directly linked to the onset of osteoporosis. Low iron concentrations may be a consequence of the menstruation process which can lead to anemia. Supplements for both calcium and iron may be recommended. Again, we suggest you consult with an expert in the field to determine what is best for your body.

PRACTICAL EATING GUIDELINES

Based on typical eating habits it is no wonder that national attention has been directed to changing the average American diet. The Food Guide Pyramid and the Guidelines for Healthy Americans were both developed to bring increased awareness of nutrition and health. Promoting and developing a diet that is high in complex carbohydrates and low in fat and sodium are all goals designed to decrease the risk of heart disease and promote general wellness. Yet, like developing an active lifestyle, committing yourself to good eating habits is not easy.

Eating out of boredom, emotional distress, and over indulging on social occasions can all under-

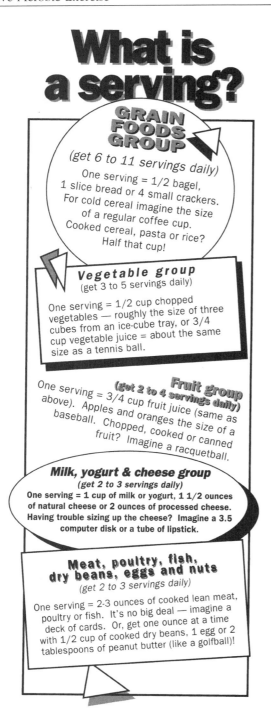

What is a serving?

GRAIN FOODS GROUP
(get 6 to 11 servings daily)
One serving = 1/2 bagel, 1 slice bread or 4 small crackers. For cold cereal imagine the size of a regular coffee cup. Cooked cereal, pasta or rice? Half that cup!

Vegetable group
(get 3 to 5 servings daily)
One serving = 1/2 cup chopped vegetables — roughly the size of three cubes from an ice-cube tray, or 3/4 cup vegetable juice = about the same size as a tennis ball.

Fruit group
(get 2 to 4 servings daily)
One serving = 3/4 cup fruit juice (same as above). Apples and oranges the size of a baseball. Chopped, cooked or canned fruit? Imagine a racquetball.

Milk, yogurt & cheese group
(get 2 to 3 servings daily)
One serving = 1 cup of milk or yogurt, 1 1/2 ounces of natural cheese or 2 ounces of processed cheese. Having trouble sizing up the cheese? Imagine a 3.5 computer disk or a tube of lipstick.

Meat, poultry, fish, dry beans, eggs and nuts
(get 2 to 3 servings daily)
One serving = 2-3 ounces of cooked lean meat, poultry or fish. It's no big deal — imagine a deck of cards. Or, get one ounce at a time with 1/2 cup of cooked dry beans, 1 egg or 2 tablespoons of peanut butter (like a golfball)!

TABLE 11-4
Nutrition and Your Health: Dietary Guidelines for Americans

- eat a variety of foods
- maintain a healthy weight
- choose a diet low in fat, saturated fat, and cholesterol
- choose a diet with plenty of vegetables, fruits, and grain products
- use sugars only in moderation
- use salt and sodium only in moderation
- if you drink alcoholic beverages, do so in moderation

Adapted from the U.S. Department of Agriculture and the U.S. Department of Health and Human Services, 1990, third edition.

---

people undermine their dietary goals by over-reacting to their food choices. If someone decides to eat a few cookies or some chips, they may feel they might as well eat the whole bag. This is a physical and emotional battle that only reinforces bad eating habits. Some snack foods such as cookies and chips should be eaten sparingly but they do not have to be avoided altogether. Give yourself permission to **eat a few** "fattening" items each week guilt free. Table 11-4 provides you with sensible eating guidelines that you can incorporate into your own dietary goals.

EATING AND WORKING OUT: WHICH COMES FIRST?

The interdependence of energy intake and energy expenditure makes timing meals and workout an important consideration. An athlete in training for an event may eat a special diet several days in advance of their competition. An endurance runner may even eat during a race in order to sustain valuable energy stores! For the average aerobic participant deciding when to eat and when to exercise usually involves asking yourself three questions:

1. How long ago was your last snack or meal?
2. How long before your next workout?
3. What has been your previous experience with exercise and eating?

In general, large or heavy meals consisting primarily of protein or fat, should be avoided for several hours prior to moderate exercise. A lighter

---

mine good eating habits. The key is to use the same tips for motivation and goal setting that keep you committed to exercise. Define yourself as a "good eater" not an "unsuccessful dieter". Balancing sensible nutrition with an occasional excess of food is possible, as long as there is a resolve to return to a moderate diet. Unfortunately, some meal or snack consisting of primarily simple carbohydrates can usually be consumed up to 30 minutes prior to exercise with positive results. Many exercise enthusiasts choose milk, a banana, apple or even a sports drink. Yet, some research indicates the foods high in acid and/or containing high quantities of fructose (orange juice, cranberry juice, etc.) have been associated with abdominal discomfort and cramping and should be avoided unless your personal experience tells you otherwise. Food that is higher in complex carbohydrates, a bagel or bowl of cereal, might need to be eaten an hour or more before exercise, depending upon your own level of comfort.

EATING DISORDERS

Struggling with food choices is something each of us does every day. We may not always make the best selection, especially when tempted with our favorite junk food. Some of us may even eat a whole plate of brownies when we originally intended to eat only a few. While this kind of behavior does not promote healthy eating habits, it is very different from having an eating disorder.

Persons who are preoccupied with becoming overweight can develop the serious eating disorders of bulimia or anorexia nervosa. Both disorders are more commonly seen in females, beginning with the adolescent and progressing through middle age. A person with **bulimia** gorges herself *with hundreds of calories and then induces vomiting*. She is obsessed with staying thin and will try numerous ways to eliminate calories including the use of laxatives and diuretics. Such abusive practices have led to liver damage, stomach rupture, heart complications, tooth decay and inflammation of the lining of the mouth and throat.

Anorexia nervosa is brought on by the same obsession to stay thin, but *is characterized by almost complete denial of hunger. The anorexic simply doesn't eat*. In addition, she is often obsessed with exercise, may abuse laxatives and even induce vomiting. Unfortunately, anorexia nervosa has severe and life threatening consequences. If left untreated anorexia can be fatal. Death is usually caused by heart complications as the heart muscle atrophies (wastes away) and can no longer sustain the heavy demands placed upon it.

Bulimia and anorexia nervosa often develop in individuals who have a poor self-concept and/or a distorted self-image. They believe they are overweight and that being thin will cure their unhappiness and actually improve their self-concept. With all the hype in the media to be thin, it is no wonder the problem is so prevalent.

There are much healthier ways to achieve a lean and beautiful body. A long term commitment to regular exercise with proper nutritional practices will give you the body you want—it just won't happen over night. If you feel a tendency to purge or starve, or if you have an obsession with becoming overweight, we strongly recommend counseling. A counselor will help you deal with the issues that are causing you to feel this way and may refer you to professionals who can help understand how proper nutrition and exercise work together. Often, a more informed approach is the answer to achieving the desired goal.

SUMMARY

A healthy body depends on regular exercise and a good diet. Realize that ignoring your diet will affect your physical performance during exercise. Be aware that choosing a rapid weight loss diet or megadose vitamins to resolve nutritional and weight concerns will not provide you with permanent results and may sacrifice your physical health and well-being. Losing weight or more specifically, fat, is the result of taking in fewer calories than the body consumes. However, taking in too few calories will disrupt normal metabolic function and not promote weight loss. Sensible eating should follow the guidelines provided outlined in this chapter. An individual whose daily diet contains a variety of foods will likely receive an adequate supply of the essential nutrients: carbohydrates, proteins, fats, vitamins, minerals, and water. With a fast-paced lifestyle, proper nutrition may be sacrificed. Your doctor, dietician, or licensed nutritionist will be the best judge of your diet and whether it should be supplemented.

GLOSSARY

Adipose Tissue—the accumulation of fat cells.

Amino Acids—small chemical chains that make up protein molecules.

Anorexia Nervosa—an eating disorder characterized by an almost complete abstention from eating and affecting those individuals who are obsessed with being "thin".

Bulimia—an eating disorder characterized by binging and purging (vomiting) food. This behavior is driven by the same obsession to be thin.

An exercise in nutrition

The exercise of eating. It's one of America's favorite pastimes and — when it's done right — it can help you look and feel great.

Building a better diet is easy. Start one "block" at a time — or, better yet one serving at a time with the Food Guide Pyramid. The Pyramid helps unlock the secret of a healthy diet by suggesting the number of servings to consume from each food group (proportionally shown with blocks). The idea is that when you eat more of the foods in the lower half of the Pyramid, you'll automatically consume less fat and more of the nutrients we need for better health.

Try this quick exercise in nutrition to test your basic Pyramid knowledge:

Q. How many food groups are there?
___ 3 ___ 4 ___ 5 ___ 8

A. If you answered five you're getting warmed up for success. The Food Guide Pyramid goes beyond the old "basic four" food groups to help you choose what and how much to eat from each food group for good health.

Q. Can you name the food groups and the number of servings needed from each?

A. The Pyramid Workout focuses on these groups:
Grain Group (bread, cereal, pasta, crackers and rice):
    6 to 11 servings
Vegetable Group:
    3 to 5 servings
Fruit Group:
    2 to 4 servings
Meat and Protein Group:
    2 to 3 servings
Milk Group:
    2 to 3 servings
Fats, oils and sugars:
    Not a food group. Included with the message "use sparingly."

Q. Why so much from the grain group? Aren't these foods fattening?

A. These foods are not fattening because most of their calories come from complex carbohydrates or "carbs." (The fattening myth stems from what goes on top!) Carbs are an important source of energy especially in low-fat diets. Stored as glycogen in the muscles, carbs are important for exercise. Grains also provide vitamins, minerals and fiber.

Q. Isn't 6 to 11 servings of grain foods a lot?

A. It may sound like a lot, but it's really not. A small bowl of cereal and one slice of toast for breakfast are two servings. A slice of bread is one serving, so a sandwich for lunch would equal two servings. And, 1/2 cup of cooked cereal, pasta and rice equals one serving, so if you have a cup of pasta at dinner, that's two more! A snack of 3 or 4 small crackers adds yet another serving. So now you've had seven. It adds up more quickly than you think!

Q. True or False — To lose weight you should eat fewer servings from each group.

A. Seems like a simple solution but this one's definitely false. The best and simplest way to lose weight is to increase your physical activity and reduce the fat and sugars in your diet. Everyone should eat at least the lowest number of servings from the five major food groups. You need them for the vitamins, minerals, carbohydrates and protein they provide. Just try to pick the lowest fat choices in each group. Go with the grain group for a low-fat energy-rich alternative that will also help curb hunger pains — just be sure to keep your toppings light!

Look at it this way

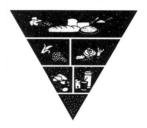

Turn the Pyramid upside down and the message becomes even clearer. Grains are an important part of any food plan. Here are six easy ways to start building your Pyramid workout with grains:

1. Wake up to carbs! Carbs jump-start your metabolism and provide energy for the day. Start with cereal, toast, bagels, muffins or waffles, add a piece of fruit and you're off.

2. Carbs to go! Stash crackers, cereal or pretzels in your desk drawer, or a bread-stick in your briefcase to satisfy hunger without a trip to the vending machine.

3. Lighten up, already! Keep toppings on breads, rolls and pasta light. Use jams and fruit purees on bread instead of butter or margarine. Try tomato or vegetable-based sauces with pasta or stir-fry noodles with vegetables.

4. Join the club! Go for the club sandwich instead of a huge Dagwood style. Use more bread and fewer fillings.

5. Recharge! Tuck a bagel or graham crackers into your gym bag to replenish the glycogen used during exercise.

6. Need a treat? Sprinkle cereal or wheat germ on your frozen yogurt, have angel food cake with strawberries or grab a handful of animal crackers. If you eat right and exercise, you can afford to indulge with your favorite dessert on occasion.

Carbohydrates—a primary source of energy for muscular work. Carbohydrates are present in foods in the form of sugars, starches and cellulose.

Complete Protein—animal products that contain all the essential amino acids.

Essential nutrients—(Carbohydrates, fats, protein, vitamins, minerals and water) each of these nutrients are necessary for the body to carry on normal life functions.

Fats—provide a continuous supply of energy to the body. Fats carry the vitamins A, D, E and K and assist in the absorption of vitamin D to help make calcium available to the bones, teeth and other body tissues. Fats provide a protective layer of insulation around the vital organs and under the skin as a means of protection against the cold.

Incomplete Protein—plant protein lacking one or more essential amino acid.

Metabolism—the mechanical and chemical processes in the body that break down (catabolism) and build/manufacture (anabolism) or convert compounds, cells and/or tissues. This dynamic process sustains growth, renewal, and waste elimination and is essential to normal body function.

Minerals—function as catalysts in numerous biologic functions including the nervous system, digestive system and the process of nutrient utilization as derived from food stuffs.

Proteins—is considered the major source of building materials for the skin, hair, nails, blood, muscles, internal organs and the brain.

Vegan—individuals who exclude all animal products from their diet and include only food from plant sources.

Vegetarians—individuals who minimize eating animal products such as meat, but may include milk and/or eggs.

Vitamins—function as catalysts in almost all metabolic reactions, regulating metabilic processes, converting fat and carbohydrates to energy and assisting in the formation of bones and tissues.

REFERENCES

Coyle, E. F. & Montain, S. J. (1992). Carbohydrate and fluid ingestion during exercise: Are there trade-offs. *Medicine and Science in Sports and Exercise, 24* (6), 671–678.

Kristal-Boneh, E. & Green, M. S. (1992). Dietary calcium and blood pressure—A critical review of the literature. *Public Health Reviews, 18,* 267–300.

Maughan, R. J. & Rehrer, N. J. (1993). Gatric emptying during exercise. *Sports Science Exchange, 6* (5).

Sawka, M. N. (1992). Physiological consequences of hypohydration: exercise performance and thermoregulation. *Medicine and Science in Sports and Exercise, 24* (6), 657–667.

U.S. Department of Agriculture. (1992). *The Food Guide Pyramid.* Home and Garden Bulletin 252. Washington, D.C.: U.S. Government Printing Office.

Wardlaw, G. M. & Insel, P. M. (1993). *Perspectives in Nutrition* (2nd ed.). St. Louis: Mosby.

The Wheat Foods Council. (1994). Nutrition Kit. Englewood, CO.: The Wheat Foods Council.

White, S. L. & Maloney, S. K. (1990). Promoting healthy diets and active lives to hard to reach groups: Market research study. *Public Health Reports, 105* (3), 224–231.

We are all sculptors and painters and our material is our own flesh and blood and bone.

–Henry David Thoreau

CHAPTER 12

Exercise and Weight Management

The attempt to lose weight has virtually become a national pastime. As many as one out of every four people are on some kind of a diet. Unfortunately, most of the weight lost by these dieters will be regained within one year. Statistics show that for every 100 dieters, 95 will be right back where they started from. And, if regain occurs in the absence of exercise, the weight gain will be mostly fat.

Methods to lose unwanted fat are numerous but generally fall into one of the following categories: dietary management, drug treatment, surgical treatment, behavior modification and/or exercise. Each of these methods has the potential to be effective, but many can be dangerous. Most fitness experts recommend the combined approach which includes dietary management and exercise. The purpose of this chapter is to show how diet and exercise, in conjunction with genetic disposition, influence weight management.

WEIGHT CONTROL

It is important to understand how the body utilizes food stuffs for energy as well as how exercise can enhance the alteration in body composition. Losing excess fat may be warranted for health reasons, or may simply be a desire of the individual. The concept of weight maintenance is quite simply illustrated below which shows that calories consumed must equal calories expended.

Energy Balance Equation

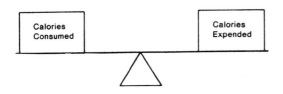

If calories consumed exceed calories expended, weight gain is the result. The opposite is true for weight loss. The concept of gaining and losing weight appears simple enough, yet, the term body weight must be examined more closely in relation to body composition. It is important to understand how much of the total weight you have lost is fat. The type of weight loss is dependent upon a complex interaction of the particular food stuffs consumed and the manner in which the calories are expended.

CALORIC DEMANDS OF EXERCISE

Calories supply the energy necessary to perform movement, but the duration, intensity and nature of the activity dictates the amount and specific source of the fuel to be consumed. Weight loss and gain is a function of caloric consumption and energy expenditure, but the overall influence of activity is often misunderstood. To be successful in managing your weight, you need to separate yourself from many popular myths about diet and exercise.

The Spot Reducing Myth

There is an ongoing rumor that performing abdominal crunches will reduce the size of the abdomen, or that trunk twists will slim the waist. Even topical creams and body massages have been credited with eliminating unwanted fat. The myth of spot reducing and other quick weight loss solutions are hard to dismiss, after all, such products are advertised on television and in magazines every day. Yet, to be successful at weight loss, the results must be safe, effective and permanent. Many solutions are temporary or simply don't work. Permanent weight loss is possible, but it requires more commitment than just taking a pill or doing one exercise. Recognizing the physical structure and

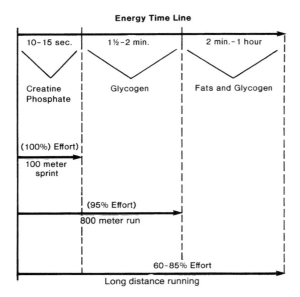

Energy Time Line

10-15 sec.	1½-2 min.	2 min.-1 hour
Creatine Phosphate	Glycogen	Fats and Glycogen

(100%) Effort)
100 meter sprint

(95% Effort)
800 meter run

60-85% Effort
Long distance running

function of the body will help you understand what activities utilize fatty acids and what exercises do not.

Isolated movements such as crunches, lunges, and leg lifts affect the body by toning muscles and increasing endurance. If additional resistance is added to any of these exercises, improved muscular strength can result. Toned muscles provide the body with definition and shape. Yet, contrary to popular opinion, *muscles unchallenged by exercise do not change into fat.* Muscle cells and fat cells form two separate types of tissue with distinct structure and function; one cannot be converted to the other—not with exercise and not with pills. However, untone or flaccid muscles are soft, lack definition and therefore may look like that of adipose tissue. Isolated exercises performed regularly have the potential to change the body's physical appearance. Weight training can even improve body composition by increasing muscle mass. Yet, isolated exercises and weight training do not have a profound affect on body fat.

About one half of the body's adipose tissue makes up a superficial layer of fat under the skin called **subcutaneous fat**. This layer is located on top of the skeletal muscles. While isolated exercises can affect muscle tone, you won't see any change if the area is covered by a layer of fat. In very lean individuals, it is possible to see muscle striations, while in obese people little tone is visible at all. The thought that exercising specific sites will target and mobilize fat consumption in that area may sound probable, but the body has different priorities. The activity of weight training is largely anaerobic, utilizing carbohydrates (glucose) as its primary fuel source. Resistance training supports

weight loss by increasing muscle mass and therefore the increasing calorie consumption during rest and activity. Yet, the thought that targeting specific areas with conditioning exercises will result in changing muscle to fat or result in consuming the subcutaneous fat located under the skin is a fantasy.

Fuel Sources During Exercise

During the first few seconds of any activity energy is derived from a substance known as creatine phosphate. When the creatine phosphate is used up (10–15 seconds), carbohydrates (glycogen) are utilized.

The next available energy source is determined by the type, duration and intensity of the activity. A high intensity, short duration activity, such as a 100 meter sprint, will continue to rely primarily on glycogen for fuel. Activities of lower intensity (60–85%) and longer duration (20 minutes and more), such as creative aerobic fitness, jogging, cycling and swimming, will derive the needed energy from a blend of carbohydrates and fats. Neither receive much of an energy contribution from protein if the participant has been eating a well balanced diet.

If your goal is to lose fat weight, the exercise or activity you choose should be aerobic in nature. For those of you who eat a well balanced diet, supplying your body with all of the necessary nutrients, you will find fat to be more readily metabolized at the lower end of your training heart rate zone. Lower intensity exercise allows the cardiovascular and respiratory systems to provide more oxygen to the body, a necessary ingredient in the production of energy from fats. The importance of proper nutrition cannot be stressed enough, because it is too often ignored. Understanding what constitutes caloric intake and how it interacts with energy expenditure is critical in the weight loss game. Only by becoming more informed about the body's physiological processes and how fat is actually stored and metabolized for energy will you be able to take control of what seems like a never ending battle with weight management.

BODY IMAGE AND BODY TYPE

Body image is the concept we have of ourselves. As described in Chapter 1, body image is an essential part of our self-image. How we perceive our body and accept certain physical characteristics, is related to our self-esteem. Evaluating your body type means observing the predominant features of your physical frame. Sheldon (1954) developed a model for describing physical body builds, characterizing three distinct types: ectomorph, mesomorph and endomorph. When examining these physical characteristics you may feel your body overlaps into two categories, but you can probably determine which one best describes your physical appearance.

Ectomorph: *Characterized by long, linear and fragile structure; small bones, long limbs, long, thin muscles with minimal muscularity.*

Mesomorph: *Characterized by prominent muscularity; large bones, thick muscles with significant definition, small waist, broad shoulders.*

Endomorph: *Characterized by round soft features; medium bones, short neck with high shoulders, soft smooth skin, in women—developed breasts, round full buttocks.*

Not only does Sheldon's model provide a means of identifying body types through physical classification, it also describes your genetic potential, or ability to alter your physical shape. Genetic factors such as the fat to non-fat ratio, type, size and number of muscle fibers and hormone concentrations are also part of your genetic potential. Each body type, as classified by Sheldon, has genetic limitations. In other words, you cannot change your basic structure, but rather, work within your genetic capabilities. This concept is important relative to exercise and explains why individuals respond differently. Just as a Clydsdale (workhorse) will never become a thoroughbred (racehorse); an endomorph will never become an ectomorph. This physical expectation lies outside the genetic potential. The underlying characteristics will always be predominant. What is important to learn is to accept your body for what it is and work within your own potential.

SET POINT THEORY AND WEIGHT MANAGEMENT

The set point theory describes the body's attempt to maintain a given body weight and prevent large gains and losses. Similar to a thermostat which fluctuates about a given temperature reading, our body weight also fluctuates about a given number of pounds. As a result of these fluctuations, the appetite control center in the brain (hypothalamus) is either stimulated or inhibited. When weight loss occurs, the appetite control center is stimulated. There is a tendency to eat more calories

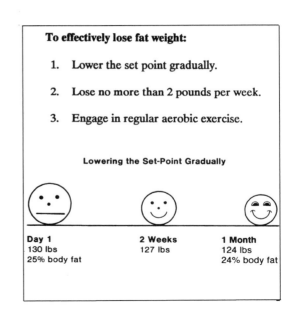

End result of rapid weight loss: Large amounts of fluids, carbohydrates and muscle protein are sacrificed for energy. Very little fat, if any, is lost. The appetite control center is turned on. The result is a rapid gain as the body returns to its set point. In the absence of exercise, much of the weight gain will be fat.

Rapid Weight Loss

Day 1	2 Weeks	1 Month
130 lbs	120 lbs.	130 lbs
25% body fat		26% body fat

To effectively lose fat weight:

1. Lower the set point gradually.

2. Lose no more than 2 pounds per week.

3. Engage in regular aerobic exercise.

Lowering the Set-Point Gradually

Day 1	2 Weeks	1 Month
130 lbs	127 lbs	124 lbs
25% body fat		24% body fat

as the body attempts to regain its original weight. When weight gain occurs, the appetite control center inhibits the desire for food and the extra weight is lost. Fluctuation in weight may also occur as a result of psychological factors, a chemical imbalance, or an illness of some sort. One of the goals in weight management is to take control of the outside influences and allow the body to function the way it was designed.

If you are interested in permanent weight gain or loss, you will need to alter your set point gradually over time, to avoid stimulating or inhibiting the appetite control center. When significant weight loss (10 pounds or more) occurs in a relatively short period of time (2 weeks or less) the body doesn't know if it's starving or simply on a diet. The physiological response to a sudden decrease in calories is the same, regardless of the reason. Rapid weight loss depletes the fat cell too quickly. As a result, the body attempts to reserve its fat stores and relies upon carbohydrates and protein to supply the energy it needs. Unfortunately, most crash diets do not adequately supply the body with carbohydrates, so when the carbohydrate stores are used up, protein becomes the main contributor.

As the diet continues, another phenomenon occurs. The appetite control center becomes increasingly stimulated. Hunger results and proceeds to protect the body from starvation. It is this stronger than ever hunger response that drives one to eat. Unfortunately, much of the body stores have been exhausted, and in the sudden rush to correct the deficit the receptor gates on all depleted cells open wide, begging to be filled. Eating becomes an obsession and the weight is gained back in a very short period of time. This is thought to be the reason why the body returns to its original weight (set point). If the weight loss occurred without exercise, then the weight which was lost in protein and fluids is exchanged for fat. The body's fat content is now greater than before the diet began. Exercise can work to slow the burning of muscle protein for energy during periods of rapid weight loss and inhibit the complete regain of fat when the diet is broken. But even exercise becomes ineffective when the body is subjected to starvation-like conditions. The only way to successfully lose body fat is to lower the set point gradually over time to avoid the body's starvation response.

Eating: A Physical or Emotional Response

Hunger *is a physical sensation that is triggered by complex chemical reactions and caused by the bodies need for nutrients.* Eating will ease this feeling. Once the physical needs for food have been met the body will provide feedback to the brain, *relieving the sense of hunger with a feeling of* **satiation**. This feedback is not immediate and eating too quickly can result in the feeling that you ate too much. Physical appetite can be suppressed by many things, including illness, medication, or stress. In some people exercise has also been associated with appetite suppression, while others find their need for nourishment increases. In addition to increased activity levels appetite can also be stimulated by temperature changes or simply the sight of food.

The sensation of hunger and eating food are not simply functions of physical need. Many people eat out of psychological desires caused by boredom, nervousness, distress, or in response to social situations. Emotional eating is a real concern for many people and is not usually conducive to a healthy diet. Eating out of boredom rather than physical hunger results in the body gaining nutrients it doesn't need. Also, the foods selected during times of emotional upheaval are not usually very nutritious. "Comfort foods" are often sweet and rich providing physical satiation that is unrelated to nutrient needs. The taste and texture of ice cream, chocolate, and other rich foods provides the body with physical sensations that are enjoyable. Frequent emotional eating can undermine dietary goals and lead to a sense of guilt or self-blame as well as weight gain. While eating for psychological rather than physical needs is a complicated issue, acknowledging its existence, perhaps even in your own dietary habits, is part of understanding overall nutrition. If you or someone you know seeks out food in times of distress, one way to curtail this behavior is to substitute it with another more positive behavior. Exercise can also be used to relieve stress. The sense of enjoyment received from food can also be gained from your favorite activity and without any residual guilt. So the next time you crave a whole carton of ice cream try going for a walk with a friend. Such strategies assist you reaching your goals and are part of developing a healthy lifestyle.

EXERCISE AND THE BASAL-METABOLIC RATE

There is a minimum level of energy required to sustain the body's normal functions during rest, i.e., the **basal metabolic rate.** The basal rate is a direct reflection of resting caloric expenditure. The higher the rate, the more calories burned at rest. The reverse is also true. A planned program of regular exercise has been shown to prevent a fall in basal metabolic rate and even increase the body's ability to burn more calories.

WHAT FITNESS EXPERTS KNOW ABOUT EXERCISE AND WEIGHT CONTROL

1. Insufficient exercise leads to an inefficient use of consumed calories. Excess calories are stored as fat, regardless of the source.

2. The normal internal mechanism which regulates appetite and hunger does not function properly in a sedentary individual. Exercise can work to suppress the appetite and actually increase the desire for "good" food.

3. Increased muscle mass and regular aerobic exercise will lead to greater calorie consumption at rest and during activity.

4. Small frequent meals contribute to an active and healthy lifestyle better than 1 or 2 larger meals. Eating a small amount of food five or six times a day helps regulate blood sugar levels, better distributes nutrients and calories throughout the day, and can prevent overeating. This coupled with regular activity will promote weight management.

5. Body composition and overall fitness are temporary characteristics. Without effort unwanted change can and will result. Adequate nutrition and regular exercise are the safest and most effective ways to maintain and influence these features.

SUMMARY

Weight management can be understood from a theoretical perspective. The challenge however, is to apply the principles that have been highlighted in this chapter to your daily life. There is no simple formula or substitute for dedication to the principles of good nutrition and a planned program of regular exercise. These ingredients are essential to achieving and/or maintaining the body weight and composition you desire. Other factors that may influence weight management such as physiological complications and/or emotional stress, may be regulated or controlled with the help of a physician and enhanced by a good nutritional program and regular exercise. Allow exercise to work for you. It's guaranteed to enhance your life.

GLOSSARY

Basal Metabolic Rate—the minimum level of energy required to sustain the body's normal functions during rest.

Creatine Phosphate—an important storage form of high energy utilized as the primary source of fuel during the first 10 to 15 seconds of activity.

Ectomorph—characterized by a long, linear and fragile structure; small bones, long limbs and thin muscles with minimal muscularity.

Emotional Eating—consuming food out of psychological rather than physical need.

Endomorph—characterized by soft round features; medium bones, short neck with high shoulders, soft smooth skin; in women—developed breasts, full round buttocks.

Glycogen—derived from carbohydrates, is stored in the muscles and liver.

Hunger—is a physical sensation that is triggered by complex chemical reactions.

Mesomorph—characterized by prominent muscularity; large bones, thick muscles with significant definition, small waist, broad shoulders.

Satiety (satiation)—the absence of hunger or feeling of satisfaction

Spot Reducing—the misconception that weight loss can be promoted through targeting individual areas of the body through isolated exercises.

Subcutaneous Fat—adipose tissue that makes up a superficial layer of fat under the skin cell.

REFERENCES

Sheldon, W. (1954). *Atlas of men.* New York: Harper and Brothers.

Wardlaw, G. M. & Insel, P. M. (1993). *Perspectives in Nutrition* (2nd ed.). St. Louis: Mosby.

White, S. L. & Maloney, S. K. (1990). Promoting healthy diets and active lives in hard to reach groups: Market research study. *Public Health Reports, 105* (3), 224–231.

Key Points to Remember

1. Accept your body. Learn to appreciate your unique physical make-up and work with the body you have.

2. If you wish to change your body weight, do so gradually, incorporating dietary management with regular exercise.

3. Avoid "crash" diets. The body doesn't know the difference between dieting and starvation.

4. Be patient! Think of your body as a figure that can be shaped and sculpted with careful planning. Good nutrition and exercise will do this for you once you make the commitment.

5. Remember, the commitment is for a lifetime!

CHAPTER 13

Common Aerobic Injuries: Prevention and Care

Parallel to the increase in sport participation is the increasing incidence of sport related injury. No matter what the activity, the potential for injury exists. Most of the injuries or conditions associated with creative aerobic exercise affect the musculoskeletal system (muscles, bones, joints) and are generally categorized as sprains, strains and overuse syndromes.

Sprains and strains are classified as **acute injuries** that *have a sudden onset as a result of some abnormal motion which twists, pulls and/or bends the body's soft tissue (muscles, tendons, ligaments).* **Sprains** *occur to ligamentous tissue which connects one bone to another across a joint.* **Strains** *occur to either a muscle or tendon which attaches muscle to bone.* Sprains and strains can be temporarily disabling but heal quickly when properly treated.

Of greater concern, and much higher prevalence, are the **chronic** or **overuse syndromes.** *These types of injuries typically have a gradual onset and may last for indefinite periods of time. The term overuse implies that a particular body structure has been subjected to too much stress.* The result is a breakdown of the body's shock absorbers. The rate of the breakdown and subsequent injury is determined by the type, volume and mechanics of the activity as well as the presence of musculoskeletal malalignment and/or imbalance. Unfortunately, continued overuse serves to perpetuate the injury, delaying the healing process, and often creates additional stress to other musculoskeletal structures as a result of compensation. A weak and painful shin can compromise the normal biomechanics of the ankle, knee, hip and/or low back simply because the impact forces must be absorbed by the unaffected structures elsewhere in the body. Knowing how to recognize early signs

and symptoms of overuse, when to modify the exercise activity and, most importantly, how to prevent injuries from ever occurring are some of the most commonly asked questions today.

Leading Causes of Overuse Injuries in Aerobic Dance

- Improper Footwear
- Improper Exercise Surface
- Improper Exercise Technique
- Improper Exercise Alignment
- Poor Strength
- Poor Flexibility
- Structural Imbalance
- Overweight

PREVENTION

The key to avoiding injury is prevention. Most of the preventative measures are simple and only require a little common sense.

1. **Proper footwear**—wear shoes specifically designed for the sport activity. Aerobic shoes should only be worn during class. They are not for walking, running or any other activity. Your shoes will have a much longer life if you save them for aerobics.

2. **Replacing worn shoes**—aerobic shoes worn 3 to 5 times/week for one semester will need to be replaced for the next term. Generally, the shoes will last 3 to 4 months but the life of your shoes is determined by how you wear them. The

first signs of stress for which discomfort or pain are experienced may be an indication that your shoes need replacing. When the shock absorbing materials in your shoes break down, your body will begin to suffer as the feet, ankles, legs, knees, etc. absorb more shock. This process contributes to overuse and can easily be avoided by replacing worn shoes.

3. **Proper exercise techniques**—Your instructor will demonstrate proper techniques in class. Be sure to pay attention and ask questions if you are unclear about what is being demonstrated. One of the greatest causes of lower leg injuries (shin splints, achilles tendinitis) is "dancing" on the balls and toes of your feet instead of using your whole foot (toe, ball, heel). All movements should allow for the full range of motion. This includes the foot. This is also a concern when stepping. With each step the whole foot should be placed on the platform, starting with the rear of the foot. Placing only the forefoot on the step increases use of the quadriceps and knees while minimizing the use of the stronger gluteal muscles. In addition, stepping down too far behind the step or too far to the side of the step places unnecessary stress on the landing knee. Good stepping technique maximizes vertical movements while minimizing exaggerated movements to the back or side.

4. **Maintain good strength and flexibility**—injuries are often the result of poor strength and/or poor flexibility. Your instructor will present exercises to enhance both strength and flexibility. It is up to you to make the most of these exercises.

5. **Variety training**—No single activity is completely without risk or injury free. A trained individual, using appropriate equipment, and a moderate workout schedule may still over time become susceptible to a chronic injury. Mental boredom resulting from performing a familiar routine may keep participants from paying attention to their form and technique. The physical repetition of using the same muscles over and over, even with the safest execution, may eventually subject a participant to a repetitive movement injury. Having a variety of activities to choose from will not only minimize the risk of long term injury but can prove mentally stimulating and a welcome break from an established routine.

6. **Taking time off**—vacations are something we all look forward to in our work schedule, but they may not be fully appreciated as part of an exercise program. Some people may feel guilty if they don't work out every day. However, individuals with a well-rounded fitness program and an overall active lifestyle should be sure to include rest days as part of their structured exercise regime.

7. **Avoid contraindicated exercises**—while many exercises are generally safe, not all exercises are safe for everyone. Individuals with knee conditions may need to limit squats, lunges and stepping activities. While those susceptible to neck or low back discomfort should strengthen the muscles of the trunk, they may need to adjust the way they perform abdominal crunches. Modifying movements by limiting repetitions, using a smaller range of motion, or by substituting safer exercises allow persons with individual concerns to personalize their program.

8. **Avoid overuse**—How much is too much? This question is not easily answered but the key to injury prevention is moderation. With such variety in exercise surfaces, (spring loaded floors, mats, wooden gym floors etc.) it is best to consult with your instructor. We recommend not more than three times a week for the beginner whatever the surface, and no more than 4 or 5 times a week for the intermediate and advanced student. Non-impact activities such as swimming or cycling are recommended on alternate days.

TREATMENT

Treatment or care for an injury will vary depending on the onset (acute vs. chronic), the type of tissue involved (muscle, tendon, ligament, cartilage, bone) and the willingness of the injured person to cooperate with the recovery process. However, there are some basic guidelines that anyone can follow.

Acute Injury Care

Ice is always used for the first 48–72 hours following **acute** injury (sprain, strain). It is generally administered 4–6 times a day for 20–30 minutes per session with the use of an ice pack. If allergic reactions (rash) or intolerance to the use of ice occurs, discontinue use and see your doctor. *Never place heat on a new injury!* Heat, in fact, should not be used at all without consulting a medical expert first.

Chronic (Inflammatory) Injury Care

With recurring or chronic injuries, use ice following the activity to reduce inflammation that may result from overuse. Better yet, rest or modify the activity. Anti-inflammatory medications, such as aspirin, are sometimes prescribed for chronic injuries when rest is not popular. All medications, even aspirin, should be taken only as prescribed by your physician.

ICE

Rest—Giving injuries time to heal is imperative to a quick and complete recovery. Some interruption in your exercise schedule should be expected and should not be ignored. The amount of time allowed for rest depends upon the nature and severity of the injury.

Ice—Applying cold treatment to injuries is considered a safe treatment for most people when used with the proper guidelines.

DO
1. Direct application of ice, such as an ice massage with an ice cup, should not exceed 15 minutes as ice is capable of burning the skin.
2. Indirect application of ice, such as using an ice bag with a towel or cloth, should not exceed 30 minutes.
2. Wait 90 minutes between reapplication.

DON'T
1. Ice should not be placed on injuries to the abdomen or chest, without the recommendation of a physician.
2. Do not apply chemical ice packs directly to the skin. Check for leakage as the chemicals can cause severe burns.
3. Do not apply ice to young children or the elderly.
4. Allow skin temperature to return to normal before placing in warm or hot water.

Compression—Support (tape or elastic wrap) can be applied to an injury area especially when mild swelling is present. Be careful not to wrap too tightly especially prior to exercise as tissue tends to swell naturally during activity as blood flow increases. Compression should not be administered while sleeping.

Elevation—Raise the injured extremity and rest on a chair or table when possible. This is especially important when swelling is present.

COMMON AEROBIC INJURIES

While prevention is the best method in avoiding injury, it doesn't always guarantee injury free exercise. For this reason, we have listed in detail the most common aerobic injuries and described each one in terms of recognition (specific signs and symptoms), causes, treatments and prevention. It would probably be helpful to read the specific signs, symptoms and causes of each of the injuries listed in the event that you or someone you know develops such an injury. Be sure to discuss any discomforts, painful conditions or potential injuries with your instructor. This table follows the glossary.

SUMMARY

Be sensible about how much exercise you do. Remember, taking time off is part of your total program. Know the leading causes of injury and learn to recognize the first signs and symptoms of overuse. Practice prevention to avoid injury. If an injury develops, notify your instructor and, if necessary, seek a medical referral. Never put heat on a new injury and be aware of the guidelines for applying ice. As you become more committed to exercise, you'll find you have very little time nor patience for injury. Have fun and keep your exercise program injury free!

GLOSSARY

Acute Injury—an injury with a sudden onset; usually of short duration when properly treated.

Chronic Injury—an injury having a gradual onset with a long duration.

Ligament—attaches bone to bone.

Overuse Injuries—used interchangeably with the term chronic.

Sprain—injury to a ligament usually resulting from some abnormal motion.

Strain—injury to a muscle or tendon.

Tendon—attaches muscle to bone.

COMMON AEROBIC INJURIES

Injuries/Conditions	Signs and Symptoms	Causes	Treatment	Prevention
Achilles Tendonitis	"Kicked in the calf" feeling, painful to touch heel cord, weakness when jumping, painful to stretch. Usually responds best when warmed before activity. In severe cases, grating sensation may be felt when flexing and extending the ankle. Tendon may appear red and swollen.	Overstretching, sudden forceful movement. Tight calf muscles. Overuse. Improper footwear. Excessive hill running or performing aerobic movements on the balls and toes of feet. Excessive pronation may cause heel cord to stretch in horizontal plane—resulting in overstretching of tissue.	Modify workout. Use whole foot rather than balls and toes. Stretch calf muscles gently. Use heat before activity and ice after when injury is chronic. See your M.D. This condition can lead to complete rupture of tendon if not properly treated.	Avoid overuse. Proper footwear. Proper mechanics. Good strength and flexibility of lower leg. Do not reach too far back with the foot when stepping off the step platform.
Anterior compartment syndrome	Chronic: aching pain in front part of lower leg. Warm, red, glossy appearance. May also appear swollen. Foot and ankle may become cold and lose sensation. Condition worsens with continued activity. Can become a MEDICAL EMERGENCY if symptoms persist after cessation of activity.	Overuse; muscles in front leg compartment become swollen and can compress nerves and blood vessels. Shin splints often precede this more serious condition.	Stop activity! Chronic conditions usually respond to rest. If circulation and/or sensation does not return within a few minutes, you will need medical attention immediately. Surgery will be needed to release the pressure within the leg compartment. If left unattended, the muscles will die as a result of no oxygen. If condition appears temporary, circulation and sensation are present, ice the leg. Do not compress the area with an ace bandage.	Treat shin splints (if present) to avoid this condition.
Blisters Common sites: heel, instep	"Hot spots" on the foot. Small fluid filled bubble.	Resulting from friction. Improper fitting shoes. May form under thick calluses.	Clean, cover and protect from infection.	Proper fitting shoes. Keep calluses shaved.

COMMON AEROBIC INJURIES (continued)

Injuries/Conditions	Signs and Symptoms	Causes	Treatment	Prevention
Bunions	Bony protrusion of the joint between the great toe and the forefoot. May also affect the joint between the small toe and forefoot. Can be very painful especially when bearing weight on the balls of feet.	Improper fitting shoes. High heels cause joints to bear an excessive amount of weight. May be hereditary.	Proper fitting shoes. Avoid high heels (females) See your M.D. if condition becomes painful. Can treat symptoms of pain with ice.	Proper fitting footwear.
Chronic knee pain "Chondromalacia"	Pain on underside of knee cap, usually worse with repeated flexion and extension. May also be painful when climbing stairs. Knee cap may produce sounds of creaking or grating during movement. Swelling may be present after activity. Note: creaking or grating sounds/ sensations may be present without pain, if so, this is considered to be the normal wear and tear with age.	Degeneration of underside of knee cap as a result of malalignment and overuse. Malalignment and overweight. Full squats (weighted) and downhill running may accelerate degeneration as excessive friction between knee cap and femur (high bone) cause a breakdown in the tissue.	Treat symptoms of pain and swelling with ice before and after activity. Avoid overuse. Modify activity—avoid excessive knee flexion/extension. Low impact aerobics may irritate this condition. See your M.D. for a proper evaluation and treatment.	Avoid overuse. Proper footwear. Do not perform full squats. Practice proper technique during exercise. Knees should always be aligned over ties. Step activities may be contraindicated.
Heat Exhaustion Common— less serious	Profuse sweating. Cold, clammy skin. Normal temperature. Faintness, paleness. Weak, rapid pulse. Shallow breathing. Nausea, headache. Exhaustion, collapse. Possible loss of consciousness.	Hot, humid weather. Poor physical condition. Mineral imbalance. Heavy exercise. Hot or poorly ventilated room.	Treat for shock. Elevate legs. Fan victim. Sponge with cold packs. Massage extremities lightly. Give water (no saline). Refer to doctor.	Exercise in a well ventilated room. Dress in layers so clothing can be removed as body heats up. Drink plenty of water before, during and after exercise.

Injuries/Conditions	Signs and Symptoms	Causes	Treatment	Prevention
Heat Stroke Less common— more serious	No sweating. Hot dry skin. Elevated temperature (106°–112°). Chest pains. Flushed skin. Strong rapid pulse. Labored breathing. Nausea, headache. Exhaustion, collapse. Convulsions. Loss of consciousness.	Hot humid weather. Poor physical condition. Direct exposure to sun. Use of alcohol. Dehydration. Mineral imbalance.	MEDICAL EMERGENCY CALL 911. Cool victim. Wrap in wet sheets. Cold shower ice tub. Place in semireclining position.	Same as for heat exhaustion. Persons who have had heat exhaustion are more susceptible to heat stroke.
Iliotibial band syndrome "IT band syndrome" The IT band is a band of connective tissue located on the outside of the leg (attached above the hip and below the knee) that helps support the lateral aspect of the thigh and knee. Common site: pain on outside of the knee	Pain develops in the lateral aspect of the knee during activities in which the knee is flexing and extending repeatedly. Pain usually begins sometime after the exercise has begun and continues to worsen, forcing the exerciser to stop. Swelling is not usually evident. Most people experience no pain during normal daily activities. The condition is triggered by repetitious exercise.	IT band syndrome is generally thought to result from a shortened IT band. During flexion and extension movements, the band slides forward and backward over other tissues of the knee joint creating friction. A tight band results in the development of more friction and ultimately produces pain.	Ice to reduce any swelling and pain. A reduction in the level of activity that involves flexion and extension movements such as squats, aerobics stepping, and sliding. Stretching of the IT band. Concentration on correct mechanics.	Proper post-activity stretching. Avoid overuse of the knee. Select a step which is appropriate for your fitness level, as well as, your height. Proper mechanics. Proper footwear.
Muscle cramps "charley horse" Common sites: calf, arch of foot	Painful involuntary contraction of a muscle or muscle group.	Fatigue. Dehydration. Mineral imbalance.	Stop activity. Massage cramp to relax the muscle. Gently stretch once the muscle has relaxed.	Drink plenty of water before, during and after activity. Eat a well balanced diet. Give your body a rest when fatigued.

COMMON AEROBIC INJURIES (continued)

Injuries/Conditions	Signs and Symptoms	Causes	Treatment	Prevention
Plantar fascitis	Pain under heel near inner arch of foot, may radiate toward sole of foot. Condition most painful when taking first few steps in the morning. Painful to stretch and worse with weight bearing.	Overuse. Improper footwear such as a shoe with a soft rather than firm heel counter. Tight calf muscles and achilles tendon cause plantar fascia to be overstretched as compensation for poor calf flexibility. Pronation; changes angle of pull on the attachments (plantar fascia) creating additional stress on tissue.	Ice for relief of pain. Modified workout. Arch support (not necessarily for individuals with flat feet) In-sole insert to add more cushion. New or different shoe model; must have firm heel counter. See your M.D. This condition can worsen quickly without proper treatment. Heel spur formation could result and may require surgical treatment.	Avoid overuse. Proper footwear. Good flexibility and strength in lower leg.
Shin splints	Aching pain in front part of lower leg. Is worse with weight bearing activity (running, jumping). Develops gradually over time.	Improper footwear. Surface too hard. Improper mechanics: "dancing" on the toes instead of using whole foot. Over developed calf muscles and weak front leg muscles. Excessive pronation. Short heel cord due to tight calf muscles.	Ice massage (8–12 min.) before and after activity. Rest or modified activity. Low-impact is recommended. If condition worsens see your M.D.	Proper footwear. Proper exercise surface. Good flexibility in calf muscles. Good strength in lower leg muscles. (Toe taps work well to strengthen these muscles).
Side ache "Stich in the side"	An ache or cramping sensation experienced on one or both sides of the abdomen or trunk. Usually occurs during aerobic conditioning and may cause enough discomfort to stop activity. Diaphragm muscle is thought to be cramping during activity.	Irregular breathing. Eating too much or too soon before a workout. Poor condition.	Slow or stop activity to regulate breathing pattern. Continue at a walking pace and raise arms above head. If pain persists, apply direct pressure.	Maintain comfortable and rhythmical breathing during activity. Allow at least two hours for digestion following a large meal.

COMMON AEROBIC INJURIES (continued)

Injuries/Conditions	Signs and Symptoms	Causes	Treatment	Prevention
Sprain Common sites: ankle, knee	Pain, swelling, disability if severe. Should be evaluated by a doctor and x-rayed to rule out fracture.	Sudden abnormal twist forces ligaments beyond normal range of motion.	I.C.E. Ice, compression with elastic bandage and elevation for 48–72 hours. Crutches are needed if limp is present. Refer to M.D.	Proper footwear. Proper technique. Avoid continued exercise when fatigued as injuries often occur in a state of fatigue.
Strain Common sites: quads, hamstrings, calves	Pain, swelling, loss of function or restricted movement. A palpable lump, bump or depression may be felt. May have felt "twinge" just prior to strain and/or heard a "snap."	Sudden abnormal movement causes muscle to overstretch. Overstretching. Muscle strength imbalance. Fatigue and overuse weakens muscles making them more susceptible to injury.	Ice massage (ice cup) 8–12 minutes. Ice pack for 20–30 minutes. Slow return to activity with good warm-up and stretching program.	Proper stretching. Good warm-up. Avoid overuse.
Stress fracture Common sites: lower leg, foot	May feel like a "shin splint pain" but is usually much more severe. Aches all the time, even at rest. Is worse at night. Weight bearing activity can cause excruciating pain. X-ray will not reveal evidence of stress fracture for 12–15 days after extreme pain is experienced.	Overuse. Use of ankle weights during weight bearing activity such as running, hopping, jumping has been associated with development of stress fracture to foot, lower leg and hip.	Complete rest from all weight bearing activity. Ice 3–4 times/day. Physician will likely prescribe anti-inflammatory medication.	Good strength. Proper footwear. Proper surface. Proper mechanics. Avoid overuse. Never use ankle weights during aerobic conditioning.

Movement provides a two-way channel of learning, being both a way to find out and a form of accomplishment.

—Department of Education and Science, 1972

APPENDIX B

Program Planning and Effectiveness

WHY USE CALENDARS AND WORKOUT REPORTS?

Many colleges and universities offer fitness classes that meet only two or three times each week. To improve your fitness level and achieve the "training effect", aerobic exercise must be performed a minimum of three days each week. By the end of the course even students who are new to exercise will want to increase the number of days they workout. By doing a variety of activities at a moderate intensity you could safely exercise as many as six days per week.

Writing down your intentions (objectives) and actions (outcomes) is one technique for monitoring the progress of your program and helping you achieve your training goals. It is very important that your actions support your goals. Detailing individual workouts allows you and your instructor to compare your actions with the established guidelines for total fitness. A variety of forms have been included to enable each student to discover the modes and methods of exercising that are compatible with their schedule, lifestyle, and/or interests.

1. A **MONTHLY CALENDAR** will help students keep track of all of their activities in and outside of class, providing an overall picture of their training schedule for themselves and their instructor. Keep the calendar in a convenient and accessible place, like on a refrigerator, so that at the end of each day an accurate record can be made.

2. A **WEEKEND WORKOUT REPORT** is a detailed account of any extracurricular exercise session. This workout can involve any level of individual or social interaction and may include any cardiovascular activity. This report is designed to help each participant recognize the overall effectiveness of their exercise session. The workout format and physical effects can be compared to the recommendations for fitness training (FITT). The psychological aspects can be used to help prepare and motivate each participant for another session.

3. An **INDIVIDUAL WORKOUT REPORT** is a detailed account of a self-initiated workout performed alone. It can involve any cardiovascular activity that can safely be performed alone. In this situation individual students are responsible for initiating a workout and then motivating themselves to continue. The assignment is to recognize the physical and psychological differences of individual exercise and how this method of activity may be an effective option within your regular workout schedule.

4. A **SOCIAL WORKOUT REPORT** describes activity performed with family and/or friends. Responsibility for motivation is shared. Again the assignment is to recognize the physical and psychological differences between partner/group exercise compared to an individual workout and how this method of activity may be an effective option within a regular workout schedule.

5. An **ADVENTURE WORKOUT REPORT** is a detailed account of a new activity. The assignment is to demonstrate that variety can be used to enhance workouts, provide ongoing motivation, and/or to develop new skills.

6. A **VIDEO WORKOUT REPORT** is each students personal evaluation of a commercial exercise video. This provides students with an opportunity to critically evaluate the contents and effectiveness of a specific video and consider the viability of using it for their own workouts.

HOW TO USE THE SELF-INITIATED WORKOUT REPORTS?

<u>ASSIGNMENT OBJECTIVES:</u> These logs and reports are designed to help you structure your workout sessions and exercise schedule. In addition, this assignment provides your instructor information about your overall workout program so that they can provide you with individual feedback. You may also use this opportunity to address concerns or questions and make general comments about your progress.

Considerations

1. You are encouraged to engage in aerobic conditioning at least three times per week in order to obtain and maintain cardiovascular conditioning. Once a baseline of fitness has been established additional workouts may be safely added.

2. You are encouraged to improve their muscular strength/endurance and flexibility by incorporating supplemental exercises into your weekly workout program in addition to aerobic training.

3. Start filling out the calendar by establishing weekly exercise goals and a fitness-related monthly goal.

4. You can record and monitor their overall exercise program on a calendar. In addition students can detail the contents of *one or more workout* session on the other forms provided.

5. In filling out the calendar include when you are exercising, how long and how hard you're working, as well as, the type of activity you perform. Use the FITT formula provided on your calendar to indicate these conditions.

6. YOU ARE ENCOURAGED TO USE A VARIETY OF ACTIVITIES IN VARIOUS SETTINGS. Why not try a new activity this week (skating, rock climbing, or a dance class). Try exercising alone, with a partner and in a group to establish how this affects your workout.

7. When filling out the Workout Reports remember to take your training and recovery heart rate. You may want to read the form over first so you know what considerations to make while working out. Also, be sure to make comments about your workout or ask questions about your program or your progress.

8. Consider this activity a tool to help you monitor your progress and establish effective exercise habits.

REMEMBER, HAVE FUN WITH YOUR ACTIVE LIFESTYLE!

AND DON'T PANIC IF YOU GET OFF TRACK FOR A WHILE . . . RE-ESTABLISH YOUR ROUTINE

THE KEY TO MAINTAINING AN ACTIVE LIFESTYLE IS NOT PERFECTION BUT CONSISTENCY.

DEFINE YOURSELF AS AN ACTIVE PERSON AND YOU WILL BECOME ONE!!!!

Name: _____

Class Day _____ Time _____

*************** KEY ***************

Frequency - record on day of activity
Intensity - record Perceived Exertion or heart rate
Time - designate how long activity lasted
Type - describe what you did
Rest - designate when you take days off
****

MONTH

SUNDAY	MONDAY	TUESDAY	WEDNESDAY	THURSDAY	FRIDAY	SATURDAY

My weekly exercise goal for:

Cardiovascular training is _____ x this week

Strength and muscular endurance training is _____ x this week

Stretching and relaxing is _____ x this week

This month my short term goal is:

_____

WORKOUT REPORT

Name _____ Days/Time Class Meets _____

Training Heart Rate Zone _____-_____ beats per minute   Date of workout _____

I.   <u>Location of your workout:</u>

II. <u>Type of workout:</u> (please circle)   by yourself   with a partner   with a group

III. <u>Type of exercise:</u> (please check all those that apply)

_____ aerobic dance   _____ jogging/running   _____ swimming
_____ backpacking/hiking   _____ skating   _____ walking
_____ bicycling   _____ sliding   _____ water aerobics
_____ calisthenics   _____ social dancing   _____ x-country skiing
_____ circuit training   _____ stepping   _____ other _____

Please describe your workout in detail (use the back if necessary):

IV. <u>Duration:</u> How long (in minutes) did you spend on each component of your workout?

_____ warm-up   _____ muscular strength/endurance
_____ aerobic conditioning   _____ stretching/flexibility
_____ cool-down   _____ other _____

V.   <u>Intensity:</u> What was your effort during and after exercising

Training Heart Rate _____   Recovery Heart Rate _____

Describe how you felt during your workout (rate of perceived exertion or RPE) and discuss how this compared to your training heart rate?

VI. <u>Personal Reaction:</u>

What were the strengths and weaknesses of your workout?

How did you feel mentally before and after this exercise session?

Please indicate any questions you have regarding fitness or health.

INDIVIDUAL WORKOUT REPORT

Name _____ Days/Time Class Meets _____

Training Heart Rate Zone _____-_____ beats per minute   Date of workout _____

I.   Location of your workout:

II. Type of exercise: (please check all those that apply)

_____ aerobic dance	_____ jogging/running	_____ swimming
_____ backpacking/hiking	_____ skating	_____ walking
_____ bicycling	_____ sliding	_____ water aerobics
_____ calisthenics	_____ social dancing	_____ x-country skiing
_____ circuit training	_____ stepping	_____ other _____

Please describe your workout in detail:

III. Duration: How long (in minutes) did you spend on each component of your workout?

_____ warm-up	_____ muscular strength/endurance
_____ aerobic conditioning	_____ stretching/flexibility
_____ cool-down	_____ other _____

IV. Intensity: What was your effort while exercising

Training Heart Rate _____   Recovery Heart Rate _____

Describe how you felt during your workout (perceived exertion or RPE).

Was your perceived exertion consistent with your training heart rate? _____

V.   Personal Reaction:

Compared to exercising with other people how did you feel before, during and after this exercise session?

Evaluate this exercise session in terms of effectiveness?

List other activities that you might enjoy performing by yourself.

SOCIAL WORKOUT REPORT

Name _____ Days/Time Class Meets _____

Training Heart Rate Zone _____-_____ beats per minute   Date of workout _____

I.   Location of your workout:

II.   With whom did you work out:

III. Type of exercise: (please check all those that apply)

_____ aerobic dance	_____ jogging/running	_____ swimming
_____ backpacking/hiking	_____ skating	_____ walking
_____ bicycling	_____ sliding	_____ water aerobics
_____ calisthenics	_____ social dancing	_____ x-country skiing
_____ circuit training	_____ stepping	_____ other _____

Please describe your workout in detail:

IV.   Duration: How long (in minutes) did you spend on each component of your workout?

_____ warm-up	_____ muscular strength/endurance
_____ aerobic conditioning	_____ stretching/flexibility
_____ cool-down	_____ other _____

V.   Intensity: What was your effort while exercising?

Training Heart Rate _____   Recovery Heart Rate _____

Describe how you felt during your workout (perceived exertion or RPE).

Was your perceived exertion consistent with your training heart rate? _____

VI.   Personal Reaction:

Compared to exercising alone, how did you feel before, during and after this exercise session?

What is the best aspect of working out with other people?

What are the drawbacks to working out with someone else?

ADVENTURE WORKOUT REPORT

Name _____ Days/Time Class Meets _____

Training Heart Rate Zone _____-_____ beats per minute   Date of workout _____

I.   Location of your workout:

II. Type of adventure planned and who went with you:

III. Please describe in detail your activity/workout (use the back if necessary):

IV. Duration: How much time, if any, did you spend on each of the following?

       _____ warm-up   _____ muscular strength/endurance
       _____ aerobic conditioning   _____ stretching/flexibility
       _____ cool-down   _____ other _____

V.   Intensity: What was your effort _____ Did it vary or remain consistent? _____

     Do you believe that this activity could be used to promote cardiovascular fitness?

     _____

VI. Personal Reaction:

     Had you tried this activity before? If so, how long ago?

     Describe any disappointments you experienced during this activity.

     What was the best part of this adventure?

     Would you try this activity again? Why or Why not?

VIDEO WORKOUT REPORT

Name _____ Days/Time Class Meets _____

Name of the Video _____ Year produced _____

I. Type of activity performed in this video: (circle all that apply)

AEROBIC DANCE   BODY SCULPTING

_____ low impact   _____ 2/bands/tubing   _____ funk dance/hip hop

_____ high impact   _____ calisthenics   _____ sliding

_____ integrated impact   _____ w/weights   _____ social dance

_____ step aerobics   _____ step & sculpt   _____ stretch/relaxation

_____ other _____   _____ other _____   _____ tai chi

                                                                         _____ other _____

Please describe the contents of the tape in detail (use the back if necessary):

II. Duration: How long, if at all, did the video spend on each of these components?

_____ warm-up   _____ muscular strength or endurance

_____ aerobic conditioning   _____ stretching/flexibility

_____ cool-down   _____ other _____

III. Intensity: How would you describe the intensity of this tape? (Circle all that apply.)

              Beginning   **Intermediate**   **Advanced**

IV. Skill Level:

How would you describe the skills demonstrated here? (Circle all that apply.)

              Beginning   **Intermediate**   **Advanced**

V. Personal Reaction:

Would this be an effective workout for you? _____ Why or why not?

Identify your favorite and least favorite aspect of this video?

How would you rate the instructor's ability to teach movements and demonstrate correct technique?

What type of modifications were shown?